ACUTE LYMPHOBLASTIC LEUKEMIA - TARGETED BIOLOGICAL IMMUNE THERAPIES

A book in the Modern Medicine Series

Kerry Atkinson MBBS MD DTM&H FRACP FRCP

About this book

The information describing the four immune targeted therapies for acute lymphoblastic lymphoma is taken from the USA Food and Drug Administration's approval label for each drug. This information is in the public domain. All other text was written by the author. Some text written by the author occurs within the FDA label descriptions: in this case, the text by the author is in italics and the section is in parentheses. All images used in this book are in the public domain and are attributed as per the requests of their creators.

Acknowledgements

I would like to acknowledge the help that I received from Jim Severino in designing the covers for this book and for uploading it for me to Kindle Direct Publishing.

Also by Kerry Atkinson

Medical books

1. Graft-versus-Host Disease. Editors, S Burakoff, H J Deeg, J Ferrara, K Atkinson. Marcel Dekker Inc, New York, 1990.
2. Clinical Bone Marrow Transplantation.First edition. Editor, K Atkinson. Cambridge University Press, Cambridge UK, 1994.
3. The BMT Data Book: A Manual for Bone Marrow and Blood Stem Cell Transplantation. K. Atkinson, Cambridge University Press, Cambridge UK, 1998.
4. Clinical Bone Marrow and Blood Stem Cell Transplantation. Second Edition. Editor, K. Atkinson. Cambridge University Press, Cambridge UK, 2000.
5. Clinical Bone Marrow and Blood Stem Cell Transplantation. Third Edition. Eds, K. Atkinson, R Champlin, J Ritz, M Brenner, P Ljungman and W Fibbe. Cambridge University Press, Cambridge UK, 2004.
6. The BMT Data Book. Second edition. R Munker, HM Lazarus and K. Atkinson, Cambridge University Press, Cambridge UK, 2009.
7. The BMT Data Book: Including Cellular Therapy. Third edition. R Munker, C Hildebrandt, HM Lazarus and K. Atkinson, Cambridge University Press, Cambridge UK. 2013.
8. Hematopoietic Cell Transplants: Concepts, Controversies and Future Directions. Eds HM Lazarus, RP Gale, A Keating, A Bacigalupo, R Munker, K Atkinson, A Syed. Cambridge University Press, Cambridge, UK. 2017.
9. The Biology and Therapeutic Application of Mesenchymal Cells. Ed. K Atkinson. Wiley/Blackwell. 2017
10. Revolutionizing Tropical Medicine. Eds. K Atkinson and D Mabey. Wiley/Blackwell Publishers Inc. 2019.
11. Asthma: Targeted Biological Treatments 2020. Kindle Direct Publishing, 2020. e-book and paperback
12. Atopic Dermatitis: Targeted Biological Treatments 2020. Kindle Direct Publishing, 2020. e-book and paperback
13. Psoriasis: Targeted Biological Treatments 2020. Kindle Direct Publishing, 2020. e-book and paperback
14. Crohn's disease and ulcerative colitis: Targeted Biological Treatments 2020. Kindle Direct Publishing, 2020. e-book and paperback
15. Rheumatoid arthritis, Juvenile Idiopathic Arthritis, Ankylosing spondylitis, Psoriatric Arthritis and Gout: Targeted Biological Treatments 2020. Kindle Direct Publishing, 2020. e-book and paperback

16. Small Cell Lung Cancer: Targeted Biological Treatments 2020. Kindle Direct Publishing, 2020. e-book and paperback
17. Chronic Myeloid Leukemia: Targeted Biological Treatments 2020. Kindle Direct Publishing, 2020. e-book and paperback
18. Melanoma: Targeted Biological Treatments 2020, Kindle Direct Publishing 2020. e-book and paperback
19. Dementia - A Caregiver's Guide. Kindle Direct Publishing 2020. e-book
20. Breast Cancer: Targeted Biological Treatments 2021. Kindle Direct Publishing 2021. e-book and paperback
21. Non-melanoma Skin Cancers: Targeted Biological and Specifically Designed Therapeutic agents. 2022. Kindle Direct Publishing 2021. e-book and paperback
22. Hodgkin Lymphoma: Targeted Biological Treatments. 2022. Kindle Direct Publishing 2022. e-book and paperback
23. Chimeric Antigen Receptor (CAR) T Cells: The second Revolution in Cellular Theapy. 2022. Kindle Direct Publishing 2022. e-book and paperback

Natural history/conservation books

24. Bird facts for everyone. K Atkinson. Outskirts Press Inc., Denver, USA. 2014
25. Birds, Birds, Birds. Kindle Direct Publishing 2020. e-book and paperback
26. A Field Guide to the Wild Habitats of Sydney Australia. Kindle Direct Publishing 2021. e-book and paperback
27. Conserving New Zealand's Endangered Species. Kindle Direct Publishing 2021. e-book and paperback
28. Conserving Australia's Endangered Species. Kindle Direct Publishing 2021. e-book and paperback
29. Nature's Wonders: Britain and Ireland. Kindle Direct Publishing 2021. e-book and paperback.
30. Nature's Wonders: Spain and Bulgaria. Kindle Direct Publishing 2022. e-book and paperback.
31. Nature's Wonders: France's Camargue, the Swiss National Park and Portugal. Kindle Direct Publishing 2022. e-book and paperback.
32. Nature's Wonders: Cuba. Kindle Direct Publishing 2022. e-book and paperback.
33. Natures's Wonders: Japan in Winter Kindle Direct Publishing 2022. e-book and paperback.
34. Nature's Wonders: India. Kindle Direct Publishing 2022. e-book and paperback.
35. Nature's Wonders: Tanzania. Kindle Direct Publishing 2022. e-book and paperback.

36. The Silk Road: Uzbekistan and Kazakhstan – A Book in the Nature's Wonders Series. 2022. Kindle Direct Publishing 2022. e-book and paperback.
37. South Africa – From the Kalahari to the Cape: a book in the Nature's Wonders series. 2023. Kindle Direct Publishing 2022. e-book and paperback.

Other books

38. Paintings 2019 – 2021. Kindle Direct Publishing 2021. e-book and paperback.
39. Ferrari Road Cars. Kindle Direct Publishing 2022. e-book and paperback.
40. Paintings II. 2022. Kindle Direct Publishing 2023. e-book and paperback.

Quotation

Saying, "Tell me great hero, but please make it brief
Is there a hole for me to get sick in?"

From the song "Tombstone Blues" by Bob Dylan on his album "Highway 61 Revisited" released by Columbia Records in 1965.

Nobel Laureate in Literature, 2016

Table of Contents

1. Author's preface

Wow! I never thought I would start an author's preface with a word like Wow, but the complexity and precision of the four medications described in this book have had an impact on me like the Space Shuttle to the Moon or any of the most glorious wild creatures or any of the great works of art (in the broadest sense of the word). The comprehensive understanding of normal human cell biology and that of its abnormal or malignant counterparts has produced a vast number of new targets for therapeutic medications. It has benefited all categories of disease but none more so than medical oncology. When I started training in medical oncology in the mid-1970s it was often not seen as a distinct speciality and was often part of a hospital's department of hematology. Then came the monoclonal antibodies, then the tyrosine kinase inhibitors, then the check point inhibitors and now engineered monoclonal antibodies and cell-mediated gene therapies. It is hard for me to comprehend that there is currently a clinical trial underway comparing two cell-mediated gene therapies in ALL. The landscape in hematology is rapidly evolving. This tsunami of new drugs is likely to increase exponentially in the coming years with major implications for health care cost and for the education of health care workers.

Please note:

i. The text of the FDA label for the drugs described in detail in this book is taken verbatim from the FDA label specific for the drug described. These are in the public domain. All figures used are in the public domain and are attributed according to the request of their creators.

ii. I have added the paragraph on Mechanism of Action of each drug near the beginning of the description of each drug, since I think this is one of the first things clinicians want to know about a new medication. This section still also remains in its original place in the FDA label in the book.

iii. I have added clinical information throughout the book to give information about some adverse clinical events caused by the drugs described. I have made clear in each instance that this information is NOT in the FDA label. I have put all such additions in parentheses and have put the text in italics.

iv. I have also put in bold font some headings in the FDA approval labels that I think are particularly important for the clinician using these drugs to be aware of.

v. There are two numbering systems in this book: firstly, that of the Table of Contents, which lists chronologically each major section of the book and, secondly, that used in the FDA approval label. I have not altered the latter. Some sections or subsections were omitted from the full FDA Prescribing Information. Thus, the numbering system within the approval labels for each of the four drugs described is not always chronological. I included for each drug all the information that was given on its FDA label. I also followed exactly the same style as used in the FDA label. For example, if text was in bold face in the FDA label, it was put in bold face in this book.

vi. This book deals only with four biological targeted immune therapeutic agents that have been FDA-approved for clinical use in precursor B cell acute lymphoblastic leukemia (ALL).

They are:

(i). Blinatumomab (Blincyto) - a bispecific monoclonal antibody directed at CD19 and CD3

(ii). Inotuzumab ozogamicin (Besponsa) - a monoclonal antibody/drug conjugate directed at CD22

(iii). Tisagenlecleucel (Kymriah) – a cell-mediated gene therapy directed at CD19

(iv). Brexucabtagene autoleucel (Tecartus) a cell-mediated gene therapy directed at CD19

2. Introduction to targeted biologic and specifically designed therapeutic agents

The five major biomedical revolutions of the second half of the 20th century are

1. The production of monoclonal antibodies
2. The discovery of DNA and how it, RNA and amino acids make proteins
3. Epigenetics and the posttranslational modification of proteins
4. The discovery of cell signalling pathways
5. The cloning of the human genome

Taken together these discoveries in cellular and molecular biology have revealed to scientists appropriate targets for new drugs and the number that have been produced in the last 30 years, and that are still being produced, has hugely enlarged the therapeutic pharmacopeia, producing treatments - even cures - for diseases that were previously untreatable. The majority of these new treatments have been derived because of much more detailed knowledge about how human cells work. They are therefore known as **biological treatments**, often abbreviated to biologics. An example of a biologic is the monoclonal antibody rituximab which reacts specifically with the CD20 antigen present only on B cells, but with no other targets.

In addition, other agents that react specifically with one, or at most, several, targets are **chemically synthesized**: an example is imatinib, which is specific for the tyrosine kinase (TK) domain in abl (the Abelson proto-oncogene), c-kit and PDGF-R (platelet-derived growth factor receptor). Another example is sonedegib, which inhibits activation of the intracellular Hedgehog signalling pathway.

The inclusion of therapeutic agents in this book (and the others in the series) is based on their specificity for a given target. For example, interleukin 2 (IL-2) would not be included since it has a range of biological activities including the proliferation of T cells, the generation of T cell cytotoxic responses and the recall of cytotoxic T cell memory. Likewise interferon-alpha (IFN-α) would not be included since its functions include antiviral activity, antiproliferative activity, NK cell activation, cytokine induction, and interferon-stimulated gene-induction activity. This exclusion applies even though each are made constitutively in the body in response to specific diseases: they are biologic agents, but their targets are broad.

This series of books – one for each disease or disease category - explains what the new treatments are, how they work and how they compare, and interact with, conventional treatment. It is important to state that no book in this series makes specific treatment recommendations for any of the diseases covered: such decisions should be initiated and reviewed by an appropriate medical specialist. Much information on each disease is available free of charge from Wikipedia (wikipedia.org), from postgraduate textbooks on each disease and from UpToDate.com: the latter website gives information for patients and caregivers free of charge but a subscription is required for more detailed information (uptodate.com). Rather, the purpose of this series of books is to give information on newly developed biological and specifically designed treatments and their mechanism of action, enabling hopefully the reader to get a handle on these extensive additions to the medical pharmacopeia. This book deals only with biological targeted agents approved by the USA Food and Drug Administration for the treatment of precursor B cell acute lymphoblastic leukemia.

A distinction is sometimes made between monoclonal antibodies (the **mabs**) as "immunotherapy", the small specifically designed inhibitory molecules (the **nibs**) and the receptor blocking agents (the **cepts**) – the latter sometimes known as decoy receptors. However, since each category of drug has been developed from the comprehensive knowledge of human cell biology discovered over the past seven decades, and as each drug in each category is exquisitely targeted to a specific epitope on a cell surface protein (the mabs), the inhibition of a specific intracellular enzyme process (the nibs), or the blocking of a specific cell surface receptor (the cepts) I prefer to combine the mabs, the nibs and the cepts in the single category of targeted biological treatments. An example from each category are rituximab, imatinib and etanercept.

A fourth type of biological targeted agents has now been FDA-approved for therapeutic use – sonidegib and vismodegib – both of which specifically target the intracellular **Hedgehog pathway** and are now both FDA-approved for treatment of basal cell carcinoma of the skin.

A fifth type of biological targeted agents approved by the FDA for treatment in a large number of different cancers are the **check point inhibitors**, which decrease the suppression of T cell activity common in all cancers, thus enabling the patients' own T cells to act against their cancer. These agents have made significant improvements in the outcome of a number of malignancies, notably in malignant melanoma

There is now a sixth type of biological targeted therapeutic agents that have been approved by the FDA for therapeutic use: chimeric antigen receptor modified **(CAR) T cells**. The first such agent – tisagenlecleucel – was approved by the USA FDA in 2017 for use in people with acute lymphoblastic leukemia. CAR T cells are an innovative cellular immunotherapeutic approach that involves genetic modification of autologous T cells such that they express target tumor antigen/s as well as a component of the T cell activation pathway – the CD3 zeta chain. T cell surface glycoprotein CD3 zeta chain, also known as T cell receptor T3 zeta chain or CD247, together with T cell receptor alpha/beta and gamma/delta heterodimers and CD3-gamma, -delta, and -epsilon, forms the T cell receptor-CD3 complex. The zeta chain plays an important role in coupling antigen recognition to several intracellular signal-transduction pathways. Upon recognition of the tumor antigen, the transduced T cells become cytotoxic and destroy the tumor cell.

CAR T cells represent the second type of cellular therapy to be therapeutically successful. The first successful cellular therapy was the use **of hematopoietic stem cells**, introduced in the late 1960s, which offered curative treatment for diseases that were not curable by any other type of therapy.

This new drug discovery phenomenon is a therapeutic tsunami which shows no sign of slowing. The pharmcopiea has increased enormously and all medical students should consider doing a Master's degree or a PhD in molecular biology. It is only by working in a cellular or molecular biology laboratory (usually combined) that one can really understand how each of these new medications work.

It should be noted that all text on each individual drug is taken directly from the USA FDA's product approval label for that drug, including the drug's generic name, its brand name, the indications for which it is approved, its mechanism of action, boxed warnings and other details on warnings, precautions, adverse events and specific patient populations. These are all in the public domain and can be accessed at https://www.accessdata.fda.gov/scripts/cder/daf/.

Only the prodct label information was take from the FDA. All images and illustrations were taken from a variety of sources. Most of these are in the public domain, but some are licensed by a Creative Commons license. Each image carries the legend written by the creator of the image as well as full attribution details required by the creator. No images were used from the FDA's product approval label for each drug.

A side-effect seen with a number of biologic agents are immune-mediated syndromes. To distinguish them from each other, a brief summary of each is given in

2. Introduction to the new targeted biologic and specifically designed therapeutic agents

Biologics and biosimilars

A **biosimilar** is a biologic medical product highly similar to another already approved biological medicine. Biosimilars are approved according to the same standards of pharmaceutical quality, safety and efficacy that apply to all biological medicines. Biosimilars are officially approved versions of original "innovator" products and can be manufactured when the original product's patent expires. Reference to the innovator product is an integral component of the approval.

It should be noted (as in the text below) that many, if not all, of these new treatments have many, and often serious side-effects, including adverse interactions when combined with other drugs.

Finally, most of these new treatments are extremely expensive ("financial toxicity"), which renders both access to them, and sometimes compliance with them, impossible or suboptimal.

Monoclonal antibodies (mabs)

Background

In 1975, Georges Köhler and César Milstein in the UK succeeded in producing a hybridoma by making fusions of murine myeloma cell lines with murine B cells. This immortalized hybridoma could produce antibodies specific for known antigens. In 1985 the FDA approved the first fully licensed Mab (Muromonab, anti-CD3 for use in preventing kidney transplant rejection. Muromonab was produced using only murine cells and thus the antibodies produced were wholly murine. Subsequently, to decrease immunogenicity of murine antibodies, chimeric antibodies were created in which the constant (Fc) portion of the antibody was human, while the variable (Fab-binding) regions remained of murine origin. After this, humanized mabs were produced in which the framework and constant regions were human, while the hypervariable region remained of murine origin. After this, fully human mabs were produced, lacking any murine component. Finally, it is now possible to produce mabs solely using recombinant DNA technology.

Mabs may be used in many different ways. This is illustrated in Figure 1 for mabs that are developed for the treatment of disease.

Figure 1

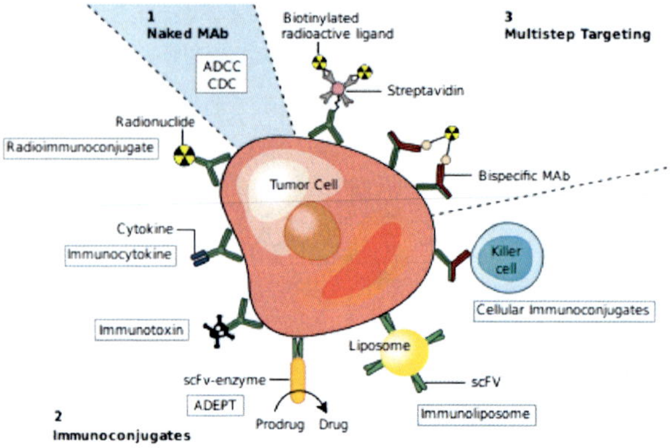

Abbreviations used in Figure 1: antibody directed enzyme prodrug therapy; ADCC: antibody-dependent cell-mediated cytotoxicity; CDC: complement-dependent cytotoxicity; MAb, monoclonal antibody; scFv, single-chain Fv fragment

Nomenclature convention for monoclonal antibodies

Murine mabs have the prefix –o- before mab; eg, abagovomab. (Note: the first murine mab approved by the FDA (Muromonab, anti-CD3) deviated from this nomenclature which was not in place at the time of its approval).

Chimeric mabs have the prefix –xi- before mab; eg, basilixumab

Humanized mabs have the prefix –zu- before mab; eg, trastuzumab

Human mabs have the prefix –u- before mab; eg, atinumab

Examples of these new agents and their mechanism of action in the treatment of non-malignant diseases

Monoclonal antibodies

- Receptor antagonists – eg, dapulimab (anti IL-4 and anti-IL13 signalling) in atopic dermatitis
- Apoptosis (programmed cell death) inducers – eg, rituximab in B cell-mediated autoimmune diseases

- Immune pathway inhibitors – eg, dipilumab for IL-4 and IL-13 signalling in atopic dermatitis, infliximab and adalimumab for TNF inhibition in psoriasis; secukinumab for IL-17 inhibition in psoriasis; ustekinumab for IL-12/Th1 inhibition and IL-23/ILTh17 inhibition in psoriasis; ixekizumab as an anti-IL17A agent in psoriasis; brodalumab as an anti-IL-7 receptor antagonist in psoriasis
- TNF pathway antagonists – eg, adalimumab for psoriasis
- Integrin pathway blockers – eg, natalizumab for Crohn's disease
- Rank ligand inhibitor – eg, denosumab for targeted treatment of postmenopausal women with osteoporosis at high risk for fracture
- Angiogenesis inhibitors – eg, ranibizumab for macular degeneration
- Dabigatran binder – eg, idarucizumab for bleeding due to dabigatran administration
- Proprotein convertase subtilisin kexin type 9 (PCSK9) inhibitor – eg, alirocumab and evolocumab for dyslipidemias
- Bi-specific antibodies – eg, emicizumab-kxwh for hemophilia A
- Monoclonal antibody-delivered toxins or drugs

A list of all monoclonal antibodies and receptor blocking agents that are USA FDA-approved for therapeutic use for either non-malignant disease, malignant disease or both malignant and and non-malignant disease is shown in Table 1 (as of December 2020).

Table 1. A list of all monoclonal antibodies and receptor blocking agents that are USA FDA-approved for therapeutic use

Generic name/brand name/type of mab	**Target**	**FDA-approved indication/s**
Abciximab/ ReoPro/ chimeric fab fragment	GPIIb/IIIa	Percutaneous coronary intervention for the prevention of cardiac ischemic complications in patients undergoing percutaneous coronary intervention or in patients with unstable angina not responding to conventional medical therapy when percutaneous coronary intervention is planned within 24 hours
Adalimumab/ Humira/ fully	TNF	Rheumatoid arthritis (RA), juvenile idiopathic arthritis (JIA), ankylosing spondylitis (AS), psoriatric arthrtitis, Crohn's disease[1], ulcerative colitis, plaque psoriasis, hidradenitis suppura[a], non-infectious uveitis

human		
Adalimumab-abdm/Cyltezo/ fully human, biosimilar	TNF	RA, JIA, AS, psoriatric arthritis, Crohn's disease[1], ulcerative colitis, plaque psoriasis,
Adalimumab-atto/Amjevita/ fully human, biosimilar	TNF	RA, JIA, AS, psoriatric arthritis, Crohn's disease[1], ulcerative colitis, plaque psoriasis
Ado-trastuzumab Emtasine/ Kadcyla/ humanized antibody-microtubule inhibitor conjugate	HER2	HER2-positive, metastatic breast cancer who previously received trastuzumab and a taxane, separately or in combination. Patients should have either: • received prior therapy for metastatic disease, or • developed disease recurrence during or within six months of completing adjuvant therapy. • the adjuvant treatment of patients with HER2-positive early breast cancer who have residual invasive disease after neoadjuvant taxane and trastuzumab-based treatment.
Alemtuzumab/ Campath, Lemtrada/ humanized	CD52	Relapsing forms of multiple sclerosis (MS) (previously approved for chronic lymphocytic leukemia but now withdrawn by its manufacturer for this indication in order to optimize its launch for treatment of MS)
Alirocumab/ Praluent/fully human	PCSK9 (proprotein convertase subtilisin kexin type 9) inhibitor	Adjunct to diet and maximally tolerated statin therapy for the treatment of adults with heterozygous familial hypercholesterolemia or clinical atherosclerotic cardiovascular disease, who require additional lowering of LDL-cholesterol (LDL-C).
Ansuvimab-zykl / EBANGA™		Treatment of infection caused by Zaire ebolavirus in adult and pediatric patients, including neonates born to a mother who is RT-PCR positive for Zaire ebolavirus infection.
Atezolizumab/ Tecentriq/ humanized	Programmed death ligand 1 (PD-L1)	1. Urothelial carcinoma for the treatment of adult patients with locally advanced or metastatic urothelial carcinoma who are not eligible for cisplatin-containing chemotherapy and whose tumors express PD-L1 or who are not eligible for any platinum-containing chemotherapy regardless of PD-L1 status, or who have disease progression during or following any platinum-containing chemotherapy, or within 12 months of neoadjuvant or adjuvant chemotherapy. This indication is approved under accelerated approval based on tumor response rate and duration of response. Continued approval for this indication may be contingent upon verification and description of clinical benefit in a confirmatory trial(s). 2. Non-small cell lung ancer (NSCLC) in combination with bevacizumab, paclitaxel, and carboplatin for the firstline treatment, of adult patients with metastatic non-squamous

		NSCLC with no EGFR or ALK genomic tumor aberrations or for the treatment of adult patients with metastatic NSCLC who have disease progression during or following platinum-containing chemotherapy. Patients with EGFR or ALK genomic tumor aberrations should have disease progression on FDA-approved therapy for NSCLC harboring these aberrations prior to receiving TECENTRIQ. 2. Triple-negative breast cancer (TNBC) in combination with paclitaxel for the treatment of adult patients with unresectable locally advanced or metastatic TNBC whose tumors express PD-L1. This indication is approved under accelerated approval based on progression-free survival. Continued approval for this indication may be contingent upon verification and description of clinical benefit in a confirmatory trial(s).
Atoltivimab, maftivimab, and odesivimab-ebgn) injection/ INMAZEB™	INMAZEB is a combination of three recombinant human IgG1κ monoclonal antibodies each targeting the Zaire ebolavirus glycoprotein (GP). Zaire ebolavirus encodes a sole envelope protein, the glycoprotein, which mediates virus attachment and membrane fusion with the host cell membranes. In addition, GP is expressed on the surface of Zaire ebolavirus infected host cells making it a target for antibodies that can mediate killing of these cells by antibody-dependent cellular cytotoxicity and/or other effector functions. The 3 antibodies that make up the combination can bind the GP simultaneously	Zaire ebolavirus in adult and pediatric patients, including neonates born to a mother who is RT-PCR positive for Zaire ebolavirus infection.
Avelumab/ Bavencio/	PD-L1	1. Adult and pediatric patients 12 years and older with metastatic Merkel cell carcinoma[2a]

fully human		2. Patients with locally advanced or metastatic urothelial carcinoma who have disease progression during or following platinum-containing chemotherapy or who have disease progression within 12 months of neoadjuvant or adjuvant treatment with platinum-containing chemotherapy[a]. 3. First-line treatment, in combination with axitinib, of patients with advanced renal cell carcinoma [a]Continued approval for this indication may be contingent upon verification and description of clinical benefit in confirmatory trials
Basiliximab/ Simulect/ chimeric	IL-2 receptor alpha chain (IL-2Rα) blocker	Prophylaxis of acute organ rejection in patients receiving renal transplantation when used as part of an immunosuppressive regimen that includes cyclosporine and corticosteroids
Belimumab/ Benlysta/fully human	B lymphocyte stimulator (BLyS) -specific inhibitor	Active, autoantibody-positive, systemic lupus erythematosus (SLE) in adults who are receiving standard therapy
Benralizumab/ Fasenra/ humanized	Interleukin-5 receptor-α	For the add-on maintenance treatment of patients with severe asthma aged 12 years and older, and with an eosinophilic phenotype
Bevacizumab/ Avastin/ humanized	Vascular endothelial growth factor (VEGF)-specific angiogenesis	1. Metastatic colorectal cancer, with intravenous 5-fluorouracil–based chemotherapy for first- or second-line treatment. 2. Non-squamous non-small cell lung cancer, with carboplatin and paclitaxel for first line treatment of unresectable, locally advanced, recurrent or metastatic disease. 3. Metastatic breast cancer, with paclitaxel for treatment of patients who have not received chemotherapy for metastatic HER2-negative breast cancer. 4.Glioblastoma, as a single agent for adult patients with progressive disease following prior therapy 5. Metastatic renal cell carcinoma with interferon-α
Bevacizumab-awwb/Mvasi/ humanized biosimilar	VEGF	1. Metastatic colorectal cancer, in combination with intravenous fluorouracil-based chemotherapy for first- or second-line treatment. 2. Metastatic colorectal cancer, in combination with fluoropyrimidine-irinotecan- or fluoropyrimidine-oxaliplatin-based chemotherapy for second-line treatment in patients who have progressed on a first-line bevacizumab product-containing regimen. 3. Unresectable, locally advanced, recurrent or metastatic non-squamous non-small cell lung cancer, in combination with carboplatin and paclitaxel for first-line treatment. 4. Recurrent glioblastoma in adults. 5. Metastatic renal cell carcinoma in combination with interferon-α.

		6. Persistent, recurrent, or metastatic cervical cancer, in combination with paclitaxel and cisplatin, or paclitaxel and topotecan.
Bevlotuxumab/ Zinplava/fully human	Clostridium difficile toxin	Reduction of recurrence of Clostridium difficile infection (CDI) in patients 18 years of age or older who are receiving antibacterial drug treatment of CDI and are at a high risk for CDI recurrence.
Belantamab mafodotin-blmf/ BLENREP Antibody-drug conjugate	Myeloma	Belantamab mafodotin-blmf is an antibody-drug conjugate (ADC). The antibody component is an afucosylated IgG1 directed against BCMA, a protein expressed on normal B lymphocytes and multiple myeloma cells. The small molecule component is MMAF, a microtubule inhibitor. Upon binding to BCMA, belantamab mafodotin-blmf is internalized followed by release of MMAF via proteolytic cleavage. The released MMAF intracellularly disrupts the microtubule network, leading to cell cycle arrest and apoptosis. Belantamab mafodotin-blmf had antitumor activity in multiple myeloma cells and mediated killing of tumor cells through MMAF-induced apoptosis, as well as by tumor cell lysis through antibody-dependent cellular cytotoxicity (ADCC) and antibody-dependent cellular phagocytosis (ADCP).
Blinatumomab/ Blincyto/ murine bispecific CD19-directed CD3 T cell engager	CD19	1. B cell precursor acute lymphoblastic leukemia (ALL) in first or second complete remission with minimal residual disease (MRD) greater than or equal to 0.1%. This indication is approved under accelerated approval based on MRD response rate and hematological relapse-free survival. Continued approval for this indication may be contingent upon verification and description of clinical benefit in the confirmatory trials. 2. Relapsed or refractory B cell precursor acute lymphoblastic leukemia
Brentuximab vedotin/ Adcetris/ chimeric, antibody-drug conjugate	CD30	1.Classical Hodgkin lymphoma[3] (cHL) at high risk of relapse or progression as post autologous hematopoietic stem cell transplantation (auto-HSCT) consolidation 2.Classical Hodgkin lymphoma after failure of auto-HSCT or after failure of at least two prior multi-agent chemotherapy regimens in patients who are not auto-HSCT candidates 3. Systemic anaplastic large cell lymphoma (sALCL) after failure of at least one prior multi-agent chemotherapy regimen. Accelerated approval was granted for the sALCL indication based on overall response rate. Continued approval for this indication may be contingent upon verification and description of clinical benefit in confirmatory trials. 4. Primary cutaneous anaplastic large cell lymphoma (pcALCL) or CD30 expressing mycosis fungoides who have received prior systemic therapy
Brodalumab/ Siliq/chimeric	!L-17 receptor	Moderate to severe plaque psoriasis in adult patients who are candidates for systemic therapy or phototherapy and

		have failed to respond or have lost response to other systemic therapies.
Burosumab-twza/Crysvita/ fully human	Fibroblast growth factor (FGF)23	X-linked hypophosphatemia (XLH) in adult and pediatric patients 6 months of age and older
Canakinuab/ Ilaris/fully human	IL-1β	Cryopyrin-associated periodic syndromes (CAPS), in adults and children 4 years of age and older including familial cold autoinflammatory syndrome (FCAS) and Muckle-Wells Syndrome (MWS)
Capromab pendetide/ Prosta-Scint/ murine radio-labelled (Indium ^{111})	Prostate-specific membrane antigen (PSMA)	1. A diagnostic imaging agent in newly-diagnosed patients with biopsy-proven prostate cancer, thought to be clinically-localized after standard diagnostic evaluation (e.g. chest x-ray, bone scan, CT scan, or MRI), who are at high-risk for pelvic lymph node metastases 2. A diagnostic imaging agent in post-prostatectomy patients with a rising PSA leveland a negative or equivocal standard metastatic evaluation in whom there is a high clinical suspicion of occult metastatic disease.
Certolizumab Pegol/Cimzia/ humanized (pegylated for longer duration of action)	TNF	1.Crohn's disease 2.Rheumatoid arthritis 3.Psoriatic arthritis 4.Ankylosing spondylitis
Cetuximab/ Erbitux/ chimeric	Epidermal growth factor (EGF) receptor	1.Head and neck cancer Locally or regionally advanced squamous cell carcinoma of the head and neck in combination with radiation therapy. Recurrent loco-regional disease or metastatic squamous cell carcinoma of the head and neck in combination with platinum-based therapy with 5-FU. Recurrent or metastatic squamous cell carcinoma of the head and neck progressing after platinum-based therapy. 2.Colorectal cancer As a single agent, EGFR-expressing metastatic colorectal cancer after failure of both irinotecan- and oxaliplatin-based regimens or in patients who are intolerant to irinotecan-based regimens. In combination with irinotecan, EGFR-expressing metastatic colorectal carcinoma in patients who are refractory to irinotecan-based chemotherapy.
Cemiplimab/ Libtayo/ humanized	PD-1	Metastatic cutaneous squamous cell carcinoma (CSCC) or locally advanced CSCC who are not candidates for curative surgery or curative radiation.

Daclizumab/ Zenapax/ humanized	IL-2 receptor-α	Prophylaxis of acute organ rejection in patients receiving renal transplants. It is used as part of an immunosuppressive regimen that includes cyclosporine and corticosteroids.
Naxitamab-gqgk/ Danyelza	Naxitamab-gqgk binds to the glycolipid GD2. GD2 is a disialoganglioside that is overexpress-ed on neuroblasto-ma cells and other cells of neuroectod-ermal origin, including the central nervous system and peripheral nerves. In vitro, naxitamab-gqgk was able to bind to cell surface GD2 and induce complement-dependent cytotoxicity (CDC) and antibody dependent- cell-mediated cytotoxicity (ADCC).	DANYELZA is a GD2-binding monoclonal antibody indicated, in combination with granulocyte-macrophage colony-stimulating factor (GMCSF), for the treatment of pediatric patients 1 year of age and older and adult patients with relapsed or refractory high-risk neuroblastoma in the bone or bone marrow who have demonstrated a partial response, minor response, or stable disease to prior therapy
Darzalex/ Zinbryta/ humanized	IL-2 receptor	Relapsing forms of multiple sclerosis (MS). Because of its safety profile, the use of ZINBRYTA should generally be reserved for patients who have had an inadequate response to two or more drugs indicated for the treatment of MS.
Daratumumab/ Darzalex/fully human	CD38	Multiple myeloma 1.In combination with lenalidomide and dexamethasone in newly diagnosed patients who are ineligible for autologous stem cell transplant and in patients with relapsed or refractory multiple myeloma who have received at least one prior therapy 2.In combination with bortezomib, melphalan and prednisone in newly diagnosed patients who are ineligible for autologous stem cell transplant 3.In combination with bortezomib and dexamethasone in patients who have received at least one prior therapy 4.In combination with pomalidomide and dexamethasone in patients who have received at least two prior therapies including lenalidomide and a proteasome inhibitor 5. As monotherapy, in patients who have received at least three prior lines of therapy including a proteasome inhibitor (PI) and an immunomodulatory agent or who are

		double-refractory to a PI and an immunomodulatory agent.
Denosumab/ Prolia/fully human	Receptor activator of nuclear factor kappa-B ligand (RANKL)	1.Postmenopausal women with osteoporosis at high risk for fracture 2.Treatment to increase bone mass in men at high risk for fracture receiving androgen deprivation therapy for non-metastatic prostate cancer 3.Treatment to increase bone mass in women at high risk for fracture receiving adjuvant aromatase inhibitor therapy for breast cancer
Denosumab/ Xgeva/fully human	RANKL	1.Prevention of skeletal-related events in patients with multiple myeloma and in patients with bone metastases from solid tumors 2.Treatment of adults and skeletally mature adolescents with giant cell tumor of bone that is unresectable or where surgical resection is likely to result in severe morbidity 3.Treatment of hypercalcemia of malignancy refractory to bisphosphonate therapy
Dinutuximab/ Unituxin/ chimeric	GD2 (a disialo-ganglioside)	In combination with granulocyte-macrophage colony-stimulating factor (GM-CSF), interleukin-2 (IL-2), and 13-cis-retinoic acid (RA), for the treatment of pediatric patients with high-risk neuroblastoma who achieve at least a partial response to prior first-line multiagent, multimodality therapy
Dupilumab/ Dupixent/fully human	IL-4 receptor-α (IL-4RA)	1. For patients aged 12 years and older with moderate-to-severe atopic dermatitis whose disease is not adequately controlled with topical prescription therapies or when those therapies are not advisable. 2. As an add-on maintenance treatment in patients with moderate-to-severe asthma aged 12 years and older with an eosinophilic phenotype or with oral corticosteroid-dependent asthma. 3. As an add-on maintenance treatment in adult patients with inadequately controlled chronic rhinosinusitis with nasal polyposis (CRSwNP).
Durvalumab/ Imfinzi/fully human	PD-L1	1.Locally advanced or metastatic urothelial carcinoma who have disease progression during or following platinum-containing chemotherapy or who have disease or progression within 12 months of neoadjuvant or adjuvant treatment with platinum-containing chemotherapy 2. Unresectable, stage III non-small cell lung cancer (NSCLC) whose disease has not progressed following concurrent platinum-based chemotherapy and radiation therapy.
Eculizumab/ Solaris/ humanized	Complement component 5	1.Paroxysmal nocturnal hemoglobinuria (PNH) to reduce hemolysis 2.Atypical hemolytic uremic syndrome (aHUS) to inhibit complement-mediated thrombotic microangiopathy

Elotuzumab/ Empliciti/ humanized	Signalling lymphocytic activation molecule family (SLAMF7, CD319)	In combination with lenalidomide and dexamethasone for the treatment of multiple myeloma who have received one to three prior therapies.
Emicizumab-kxwh/ Hemlibra/ humanized bispecific	Factor IXa, Factor X (bridges activated factor IX and factor X to restore the function of missing activated factor VIII that is needed for effective hemostasis)	Routine prophylaxis to prevent or reduce the frequency of bleeding episodes in adult and pediatric patients ages newborn and older with hemophilia A (congenital factor VIII deficiency) with or without factor VIII inhibitors.
Eptinezumab-jjmr/VYEPTI/ humanized	CGRP	VYEPTI is a calcitonin gene-related peptide antagonist indicated for the preventive treatment of migraine in adults. Eptinezumab-jjmr is a humanized monoclonal antibody that binds to calcitonin gene-related peptide (CGRP) ligand and blocks its binding to the receptor
Erenumab-aooe/Aimovig/ fully human	Calcitonin gene-related peptide receptor (CGRP receptor)	Antagonist indicated for the preventive treatment of migraine in adults
Evolocumab/ Repatha/fully human	Proprotein convertase subtilisin kexin type 9 (PCSK9)	1. To reduce the risk of myocardial infarction, stroke, and coronary revascularization in adults with established cardiovascular disease. 2. As an adjunct to diet, alone or in combination with other lipid-lowering therapies (e.g., statins, ezetimibe), for treatment of adults with primary hyperlipidemia (including heterozygous familial hypercholesterolemia) to reduce low-density lipoprotein cholesterol (LDL-C). 3. As an adjunct to diet and other LDL-lowering therapies (e.g., statins, ezetimibe, LDL apheresis) in patients with homozygous familial hypercholesterolemia (HoFH) who require additional lowering of LDL-C.
Gemtuzumab ozogamicin/ Mylotarg/ humanized antibody-drug conjugate (N-acetyl gamma calichea-micin)	CD33	1.Newly-diagnosed CD33-positive acute myeloid leukemia (AML) in adults 2.Relapsed or refractory CD33-positive AML in adults and in pediatric patients 2 years and older
Golimumab/ Simponi/fully	TNF	1.Moderately to severely active RA in adults, in combination with methotrexate

human		2.Active psoriatic arthritis in adults, alone or in combination with methotrexate 3.Active AS in adults
Golimumab/ Simponi Aria/ fully human	TNF	1.Moderately to severely RA in combination with methotrexate 2.Active psoriatic arthritis 3.Active AS
Guselkumab/ Tremfya/fully human	IL-23	Adult patients with moderate-to-severe plaque psoriasis who are candidates for systemic therapy or phototherapy
Ibalizumab-uiyk/Trogarzo/ humanized	CD4	In combination with other antiretroviral(s), for the treatment of human immunodeficiency virus type 1 (HIV-1) infection in heavily treatment-experienced adults with multidrug resistant HIV-1 infection failing their current antiretroviral regimen
Ibritumomab tiuxetan/ Zevalin/ murine radio-immunoconjug-ate (the chelate tiuxetan, which tightly binds to $Indium^{111}$ or $Ytrium^{90}$, is covalently linked to ibritumomab. The beta emission from Y^{90} induces cellular damage by the formation of free radicals in the target and neighboring cells)	CD20	1.Relapsed or refractory, low-grade or follicular B cell non-Hodgkin's lymphoma 2. Previously untreated follicular B cell non-Hodgkin lymphoma who achieve a partial or complete response to first-line chemotherapy
Idarucizumab/ Praxbind/ humanized fab fragment	Dabigatran (Pradaxa)	Patients treated with Pradaxa® when reversal of the anticoagulant effects of dabigatran is needed: 1. For emergency surgery/urgent procedures 2. In life-threatening or uncontrolled bleeding. This indication is approved under accelerated approval based on a reduction in unbound dabigatran and normalization of coagulation parameters in healthy volunteers. Continued approval for this indication may be contingent upon the results of an ongoing cohort case series study.

Inebilizumab-cdon/ UPLIZNATM	CD19	UPLIZNA is a CD19-directed cytolytic antibody indicated for the treatment of neuromyelitis optica spectrum disorder (NMOSD) in adult patients who are anti-aquaporin-4 (AQP4) antibody positive.
Infliximab/ Remicade/ chimeric	TNF-α	1. Crohn's disease for reducing signs and symptoms and inducing and maintaining clinical remission in adult patients with moderately to severely active disease who have had an inadequate response to conventional therapy. For reducing the number of draining enterocutaneous and rectovaginal fistulas and maintaining fistula closure in adult patients with fistulizing disease. 2. Pediatric Crohn's disease for reducing signs and symptoms and inducing and maintaining clinical remission in pediatric patients with moderately to severely active disease who have had an inadequate response to conventional therapy. 3.Ulcerative colitis for reducing signs and symptoms, inducing and maintaining clinical remission and mucosal healing, and eliminating corticosteroid use in adult patients with moderately to severely active disease who have had an inadequate response to conventional therapy. 4. Pediatric ulcerative colitis for reducing signs and symptoms and inducing and maintaining clinical remission in pediatric patients with moderately to severely active disease who have had an inadequate response to conventional therapy. 5. Rheumatoid arthritis in combination with methotrexate for reducing signs and symptoms, inhibiting the progression of structural damage, and improving physical function in patients with moderately to severely active disease. 6. Ankylosing spondylitis for reducing signs and symptoms in patients with active disease. 7. Psoriatic arthritis for reducing signs and symptoms of active arthritis, inhibiting the progression of structural damage, and improving physical function. 8. Plaque psoriasis for treatment of adult patients with chronic severe (i.e., extensive and /or disabling) plaque psoriasis who are candidates for systemic therapy and when other systemic therapies are medically less appropriate.
Infliximab-abda/Renflexis /chimeric biosimilar	TNF-α	Similar to Remicade: see https://www.accessdata.fda.gov/drugsatfda_docs/label/2017/761054orig1s000lbl.pdf
Infliximab-dyyb/Inflectra/ chimeric biosimilar	TNF-α	Similar to Remicade. See https://www.accessdata.fda.gov/drugsatfda_docs/label/2016/125544s000lbl.pdf

Infliximab-qbtx/Ixifi chimeric biosimilar	TNF-α	Similar to Remicade. See https://www.accessdata.fda.gov/drugsatfda_docs/label/2017/761072s000lbl.pdf
Inotuzumab ozogamicin/ Besponsa/ humanized; antibody-drug conjugate (N-acetyl gamma calicheamicin)	CD22	Adults with relapsed or refractory B cell precursor acute lymphoblastic leukemia (ALL)
Ipilimomab/ Yervoy/fully human	CTLA-4	Melanoma • Treatment of unresectable or metastatic melanoma in adults and pediatric patients (12 years and older). • Adjuvant treatment of patients with cutaneous melanoma with pathologic involvement of regional lymph nodes of more than 1 mm who have undergone complete resection, including total lymphadenectomy. Renal Cell Carcinoma (RCC) • Treatment of patients with intermediate or poor-risk, previously untreated advanced renal cell carcinoma, in combination with nivolumab. Colorectal Cancer • Treatment of adult and pediatric patients 12 years of age and older with microsatellite instability-high (MSI-H) or mismatch repair deficient (dMMR) metastatic colorectal cancer that has progressed following treatment with a fluoropyrimidine, oxaliplatin, and irinotecan, in combination with nivolumab. • This indication is approved under accelerated approval based on overall response rate and duration of response. Continued approval for this indication may be contingent upon verification and description of clinical benefit in confirmatory trials. Hepatocellular Carcinoma • Treatment of patients with hepatocellular carcinoma who have been previously treated with sorafenib, in combination with nivolumab. This indication is approved under accelerated approval based on overall response rate and duration of response. Continued approval for this indication may be contingent upon verification and description of clinical benefit in confirmatory trials. Non-Small Cell Lung Cancer (NSCLC)

		• Treatment of adult patients with metastatic non-small cell lung cancer expressing PD-L1 (≥1%) as determined by an FDA-approved test, with no EGFR or ALK genomic tumor aberrations, as first-line treatment in combination with nivolumab. • Treatment of adult patients with metastatic or recurrent non-small cell lung cancer with no EGFR or ALK genomic tumor aberrations as first-line treatment, in combination with ipilimumab and 2 cycles of platinum-doublet chemotherapy
Ixekizumab/ Taltz/ humanized	IL-17A antagonist (often referred to as IL-17)	Adults with 1. Moderate-to-severe plaque psoriasis who are candidates for systemic therapy or phototherapy. 2. Active psoriatic arthritis. 3. Active ankylosing spondylitis
Margetuximab-cmkb/ Margenza	Her2/neu	Margenza is a HER2/neu receptor antagonist indicated, in combination with chemotherapy, for the treatment of adult patients with metastatic HER2 positive breast cancer who have received two or more prior anti-HER2 regimens, at least one of which was for metastatic disease
Mepolizumab/ Nucala/ humanized	IL-5	Add-on maintenance treatment of patients with severe asthma aged 12 years and older, and with an eosinophilic phenotype
Mogamuliz-umab/ Poteligeo/ humanized	CCR4 (CC chemo-kines have 2 adjacent cysteine near their amino terminus)	Adult patients with relapsed or refractory mycosis fungoides or Sézary syndrome after at least one prior systemic therapy
Moxetumomab pasudotox Lumoxiti/ murine antibody-drug conjugate. (the toxin called PE38, is a 38kDa fragment of Pseudomonas exotoxin A.	CD22	Adult patients with relapsed or refractory hairy cell leukemia (HCL) who received at least two prior systemic therapies, including treatment with a purine nucleoside analog (PNA)
Natalizumab/ Tysabri/ humanized	α4 integrin	1. Multiple sclerosis (MS): as monotherapy for the treatment of patients with relapsing forms of multiple sclerosis to delay the accumulation of physical disability and reduce the frequency of clinical exacerbations. TYSABRI is generally recommended for patients who have had an inadequate response to, or are unable to tolerate, an alternate MS therapy.

		2.Crohn's disease: inducing and maintaining clinical response and remission in adult patients with moderately to severely active Crohn's disease with evidence of inflammation who have had an inadequate response to, or are unable to tolerate, conventional Crohn's disease therapies and inhibitors of TNF-α.
Necitumumab/ Portrazza/ fully human	EGFR	In combination with gemcitabine and cisplatin, for first-line treatment of patients with metastatic squamous non-small cell lung cancer
Nivolumab/ Opdivo/ fully human	PD-1	Melanoma • patients with unresectable or metastatic melanoma, as a single agent or in combination with ipilimumab • patients with melanoma with lymph node involvement or metastatic disease who have undergone complete resection, in the adjuvant setting. Non-Small Cell Lung Cancer (NSCLC) • adult patients with metastatic non-small cell lung cancer expressing PD-L1 (≥1%) as determined by an FDA-approved test, with no EGFR or ALK genomic tumor aberrations, as first-line treatment in combination with ipilimumab. • adult patients with metastatic or recurrent non-small cell lung cancer with no EGFR or ALK genomic tumor aberrations as first-line treatment, in combination with ipilimumab and 2 cycles of platinum-doublet chemotherapy. • patients with metastatic non-small cell lung cancer and progression on or after platinum-based chemotherapy. Patients with EGFR or ALK genomic tumor aberrations should have disease progression on FDA-approved therapy for these aberrations prior to receiving OPDIVO . Malignant Pleural Mesothelioma • adult patients with unresectable malignant pleural mesothelioma, as first-line treatment in combination with ipilimumab. Renal Cell Carcinoma (RCC) • patients with intermediate or poor risk advanced renal cell carcinoma, as a first-line treatment in combination with ipilimumab. • patients with advanced renal cell carcinoma, as a first-line treatment in combination with cabozantinib. • patients with advanced renal cell carcinoma who have received prior antiangiogenic therapy. Classical Hodgkin Lymphoma (cHL)

		• adult patients with classical Hodgkin lymphoma that has relapsed or progressed after • autologous hematopoietic stem cell transplantation (HSCT) and brentuximab vedotin, or • 3 or more lines of systemic therapy that includes autologous HSCT. Squamous Cell Carcinoma of the Head and Neck (SCCHN) • patients with recurrent or metastatic squamous cell carcinoma of the head and neck with disease progression on or after a platinum-based therapy. Urothelial Carcinoma • patients with locally advanced or metastatic urothelial carcinoma • have disease progression during or following platinum-containing chemotherapy • have disease progression within 12 months of neoadjuvant or adjuvant treatment with platinum-containing chemotherapy. Colorectal Cancer • adult and pediatric (12 years and older) patients with microsatellite instability-high (MSI-H) or mismatch repair deficient (dMMR) metastatic colorectal cancer that has progressed following treatment with a fluoropyrimidine, oxaliplatin, and irinotecan, as a single agent or in combination with ipilimumab. Hepatocellular Carcinoma (HCC) • patients with hepatocellular carcinoma who have been previously treated with sorafenib, as a single agent or in combination with ipilimumab. Esophageal Squamous Cell Carcinoma (ESCC) • patients with unresectable advanced, recurrent or metastatic esophageal squamous cell carcinoma after prior fluoropyrimidine- and platinum-based chemotherapy. This indication is approved under accelerated approval based on overall response rate and duration of response. Continued approval for this indication may be contingent upon verification and description of clinical benefit in confirmatory trials.
Obiltoxaximab/ Anthim/ chimeric	Protective antigen of the Anthrax toxin	Adult and pediatric patients for treatment of inhalational anthrax due to B. anthracis in combination with appropriate antibacterial drugs and, for prophylaxis of inhalational anthrax when alternative therapies are not available or are not appropriate.

Obinutuzumab /Gazyva/ humanized	CD20	1.In combination with chlorambucil, for the treatment of patients with previously untreated chronic lymphocytic leukemia 2. In combination with bendamustine followed by GAZYVA monotherapy, for the treatment of patients with follicular lymphoma who relapsed after, or are refractory to, a rituximab-containing regimen. 3. In combination with chemotherapy followed by GAZYVA monotherapy in patients achieving at least a partial remission, for the treatment of adult patients with previously untreated stage II bulky, III or IV follicular lymphoma.
Ocrelizumab/ Ocrevus/ humanized	CD20	Relapsing or primary progressive forms of multiple sclerosis
Ofatumumab/ Arzerra/fully human	CD20	Chronic lymphocytic leukemia (CLL) refractory to fludarabine and alemtuzumab.
Olaratumab/ Lartruvo/fully human	PDGFR-α	In combination with doxorubicin, for the treatment of adult patients with soft tissue sarcoma (STS) with a histologic subtype for which an anthracycline-containing regimen is appropriate and which is not amenable to curative treatment with radiotherapy or surgery. This indication is approved under accelerated approval. Continued approval for this indication may be contingent upon verification and description of clinical benefit in the confirmatory trial
Omalizumab/ Xolair/ humanized	IgE	1.Moderate to severe persistent asthma in patients 6 years of age and older with a positive skin test or in vitro reactivity to a perennial aeroallergen and symptoms that are inadequately controlled with inhaled corticosteroids 2.Chronic idiopathic urticaria in adults and adolescents 12 years of age and older who remain symptomatic despite H1 antihistamine treatment
Palivizumab/ Synagis/ humanized	F protein of respiratory syncytial virus (RSV)	Prevention of serious lower respiratory tract disease caused by RSV in children at high risk of RSV disease. Notes 1. Safety and efficacy were established in children with bronchopulmonary dysplasia (BPD), infants with a history of premature birth (less than or equal to 35 weeks gestational age), and children with hemodynamically significant congenital heart disease (CHD). 2.The safety and efficacy of Synagis have not been established for treatment of RSV disease
Panitumumab/ Vectibix/ fully human	EGFR	As a single agent for the treatment of metastatic colorectal carcinoma with disease progression on or following fluoropyrimidine, oxaliplatin, and irinotecan chemotherapy regimens. Approval is based on progression-free survival;

		no data demonstrate an improvement in disease-related symptoms or increased survival with Vectibix. Notes 1. Retrospective subset analyses of metastatic colorectal cancer trials have not shown a treatment benefit for Vectibix in patients whose tumors had KRAS mutations in codon 12 or 13. 2.Use of Vectibix is not recommended for the treatment of colorectal cancer with these mutations
Pembrolizumab/ Keytruda/ fully human	PD-1	Melanoma • for the treatment of patients with unresectable or metastatic melanoma. • for the adjuvant treatment of patients with melanoma with involvement of lymph node(s) following complete resection. Non-Small Cell Lung Cancer (NSCLC) • in combination with pemetrexed and platinum chemotherapy, as first-line treatment of patients with metastatic nonsquamous NSCLC, with no EGFR or ALK genomic tumor aberrations. • in combination with carboplatin and either paclitaxel or paclitaxel protein-bound, as first-line treatment of patients with metastatic squamous NSCLC. • as a single agent for the first-line treatment of patients with NSCLC expressing PD-L1 [Tumor Proportion Score (TPS) ≥1%] as determined by an FDA-approved test, with no EGFR or ALK genomic tumor aberrations, and is: o stage III where patients are not candidates for surgical resection or definitive chemoradiation, or o metastatic. • as a single agent for the treatment of patients with metastatic NSCLC whose tumors express PD-L1 (TPS ≥1%) as determined by an FDA-approved test, with disease progression on or after platinum-containing chemotherapy. Patients with EGFR or ALK genomic tumor aberrations should have disease progression on FDA-approved therapy for these aberrations prior to receiving KEYTRUDA. Small Cell Lung Cancer (SCLC) • for the treatment of patients with metastatic SCLC with disease progression on or after platinum-based chemotherapy and at least one other prior line of therapy. Head and Neck Squamous Cell Cancer (HNSCC)

		• in combination with platinum and FU for the first-line treatment of patients with metastatic or with unresectable, recurrent HNSCC. • as a single agent for the first-line treatment of patients with metastatic or with unresectable, recurrent HNSCC whose tumors express PD-L1 [Combined Positive Score (CPS) ≥1] as determined by an FDA-approved test. • as a single agent for the treatment of patients with recurrent or metastatic HNSCC with disease progression on or after platinum-containing chemotherapy. Classical Hodgkin Lymphoma (cHL) • for the treatment of adult patients with relapsed or refractory cHL. • for the treatment of pediatric patients with refractory cHL, or cHL that has relapsed after 2 or more lines of therapy. Primary Mediastinal Large B-Cell Lymphoma (PMBCL) • for the treatment of adult and pediatric patients with refractory PMBCL, or who have relapsed after 2 or more prior lines of therapy. • Limitations of Use: KEYTRUDA is not recommended for treatment of patients with PMBCL who require urgent cytoreductive therapy. Urothelial Carcinoma • for the treatment of patients with locally advanced or metastatic urothelial carcinoma who are not eligible for cisplatin-containing chemotherapy and whose tumors express PD-L1 [Combined Positive Score (CPS) ≥10] as determined by an FDA-approved test, or in patients who are not eligible for any platinum-containing chemotherapy regardless of PD-L1 status. • for the treatment of patients with locally advanced or metastatic urothelial carcinoma who have disease progression during or following platinum-containing chemotherapy or within 12 months of neoadjuvant or adjuvant treatment with platinum-containing chemotherapy. • for the treatment of patients with Bacillus Calmette-Guerin (BCG)-unresponsive, high-risk, non-muscle invasive bladder cancer (NMIBC) with carcinoma in situ (CIS) with or without papillary tumors who are ineligible for or have elected not to undergo cystectomy. Microsatellite Instability-High or Mismatch Repair Deficient Cancer

		• for the treatment of adult and pediatric patients with unresectable or metastatic, microsatellite instability-high (MSI-H) or mismatch repair deficient (dMMR) o solid tumors that have progressed following prior treatment and who have no satisfactory alternative treatment options,1 or o colorectal cancer that has progressed following treatment with a fluoropyrimidine, oxaliplatin, and irinotecan. • Limitations of Use: The safety and effectiveness of KEYTRUDA in pediatric patients with MSI-H central nervous system cancers have not been established. Microsatellite Instability-High or Mismatch Repair Deficient Colorectal Cancer (CRC) • for the first-line treatment of patients with unresectable or metastatic MSI-H or dMMR colorectal cancer (CRC). Gastric Cancer • for the treatment of patients with recurrent locally advanced or metastatic gastric or gastroesophageal junction adenocarcinoma whose tumors express PD-L1 [Combined Positive Score (CPS) ≥1] as determined by an FDA-approved test, with disease progression on or after 2 or more prior lines of therapy including fluoropyrimidine- and platinum-containing chemotherapy and if appropriate, HER2/neu-targeted therapy. Esophageal Cancer • for the treatment of patients with locally advanced or metastatic esophageal or gastroesophageal junction (GEJ) (tumors with epicenter 1 to 5 centimeters above the GEJ) carcinoma that is not amenable to surgical resection or definitive chemoradiation either: o in combination with platinum- and fluoropyrimidine-based chemotherapy, or o as a single agent after one or more prior lines of systemic therapy for patients with tumors of squamous cell histology that express PD-L1 (CPS ≥10) as determined by an FDA-approved test. Cervical Cancer • for the treatment of patients with recurrent or metastatic cervical cancer with disease progression on or after chemotherapy whose tumors express PD-L1 [Combined Positive Score (CPS) ≥1] as determined by an FDA-approved test. Hepatocellular Carcinoma (HCC)

		• for the treatment of patients with HCC who have been previously treated with sorafenib. Merkel Cell Carcinoma (MCC) • for the treatment of adult and pediatric patients with recurrent locally advanced or metastatic Merkel cell carcinoma. Renal Cell Carcinoma (RCC) • in combination with axitinib, for the first-line treatment of patients with advanced RCC. Endometrial Carcinoma • in combination with lenvatinib, for the treatment of patients with advanced endometrial carcinoma that is not MSI-H or dMMR, who have disease progression following prior systemic therapy and are not candidates for curative surgery or radiation. Tumor Mutational Burden-High (TMB-H) Cancer • for the treatment of adult and pediatric patients with unresectable or metastatic tumor mutational burden-high (TMB-H) ≥10 mutations/megabase (mut/Mb)] solid tumors, as determined by an FDA-approved test, that have progressed following prior treatment and who have no satisfactory alternative treatment options. • Limitations of Use: The safety and effectiveness of KEYTRUDA in pediatric patients with TMB-H central nervous system cancers have not been established. Cutaneous Squamous Cell Carcinoma (cSCC) • for the treatment of patients with recurrent or metastatic cutaneous squamous cell carcinoma that is not curable by surgery or radiation. Triple-Negative Breast Cancer (TNBC) • in combination with chemotherapy, for the treatment of patients with locally recurrent unresectable or metastatic TNBC whose tumors express PD-L1 [Combined Positive Score (CPS) ≥10] as determined by an FDA approved test. Adult Indications: additional dosing regimen of 400 mg every 6 Weeks • for use at an additional recommended dosage of 400 mg every 6 weeks for all approved adult indications. This indication is approved under accelerated approval based on tumor response rate and durability of response. Continued approval for this indication may be contingent upon verification and description of clinical benefit in the confirmatory trials.

Pertuzumab/ Perjeta/ humanized	HER2/neu	In combination with trastuzumab and docetaxel for the treatment of patients with HER2-positive metastatic breast cancer who have not received prior anti-HER2 therapy or chemotherapy for metastatic disease.
Polatuzumab vedotin/Polivy/ Humanized antibody-drug conjugate	CD79	In combination with bendamustine and a rituximab product for the treatment of adult patients with relapsed or refractory diffuse large B cell lymphoma, not otherwise specified, after at least two prior therapies
Ramucirumab/ Cyramza/ fully human	VEGFR2	1. As a single agent or in combination with paclitaxel, for treatment of advanced gastric or gastro-esophageal junction adenocarcinoma, with disease progression on or after prior fluoropyrimidine- or platinum-containing chemotherapy. 2. In combination with docetaxel, for treatment of metastatic non-small cell lung cancer with disease progression on or after platinum-based chemotherapy. Patients with EGFR or ALK genomic tumor aberrations should have disease progression on FDA-approved therapy for these aberrations prior to receiving CYRAMZA
Ranibizumab/ Lucentis/ humanized	VEGFR1, VEGFR2	1. Neovascular (wet) age-related macular degeneration (AMD) 2. Macular edema following retinal vein occlusion (RVO) 3. Diabetic macular edema (DME)
Raxibacumab/ fully human	Protective antigen of Bacillus anthracis[6]	Raxibacumab is indicated for the treatment of adult and pediatric patients with inhalational anthrax due to Bacillus anthracis in combination with appropriate antibacterial drugs, and for prophylaxis of inhalational anthrax when alternative therapies are not available or are not appropriate. Limitations of use: • The effectiveness of raxibacumab is based solely on efficacy studies in animal models of inhalational anthrax. • There have been no studies of raxibacumab in the pediatric population. Dosing in pediatric patients was derived using a population PK approach. • Raxibacumab does not cross the blood-brain barrier and does not prevent or treat meningitis. Raxibacumab should be used in combination with appropriate antibacterial drug
Reslizumab/ Cinqair/ humanized	IL-5	Add-on maintenance treatment of patients with severe asthma aged 18 years and older, and with an eosinophilic phenotype. Limitations of use: CINQAIR is not indicated for • treatment of other eosinophilic conditions • relief of acute bronchospasm or status asthmaticus

Rituximab/ Rituxan/ chimeric	CD20	1. Non-Hodgkin's lymphoma o Relapsed or refractory, low grade or follicular, CD20-positive B as a single agent. o Previously untreated follicular, CD20-positive, B cell in combination with first line chemotherapy and, in patients achieving a complete or partial response to RITUXAN in combination with chemotherapy, as single-agent maintenance therapy. o Non-progressing (including stable disease), low-grade, CD20 positive, B cell as a single agent after first-line cyclophosphamide, vincristine, and prednisone (CVP) chemotherapy. o Previously untreated diffuse large B cell, CD20-positive in combination with (cyclophosphamide, doxorubicin, vincristine, and prednisone) (CHOP) or other anthracycline-based chemotherapy regimens. 2. Chronic lymphocytic leukemia (CLL) o Previously untreated and previously treated CD20 positive CLL in combination with fludarabine and cyclophosphamide (FC). 3. Rheumatoid arthritis (RA) in combination with methotrexate in adult patients with moderately-to severely-active RA who have inadequate response to one or more TNF antagonist therapies 4. Granulomatosis with polyangiitis (GPA) (Wegener's granulomatosis) and microscopic polyangiitis (MPA) in adult patients in combination with glucocorticoids 5. Moderate to severe pemphigus vulgaris (PV) in adult patients
Rituximab and hyaluronidase/ chimeric co-formulated with hyaluronidase (a human endoglycos-idase)	CD20	1. Follicular lymphoma (FL) o Relapsed or refractory, follicular lymphoma as a single agent o Previously untreated follicular lymphoma in combination with first line chemotherapy and, in patients achieving a complete or partial response to rituximab in combination with chemotherapy, as single agent maintenance therapy o Non-progressing (including stable disease), follicular lymphoma as a single agent after first-line cyclophosphamide, vincristine, and prednisone (CVP) chemotherapy 2. Diffuse large B cell lymphoma (DLBCL) o Previously untreated diffuse large B cell lymphoma in combination with cyclophosphamide, doxorubicin, vincristine, prednisone (CHOP) or other anthracycline-based chemotherapy regimens 3. Chronic lymphocytic leukemia (CLL)

		o Previously untreated and previously treated CLL in combination with fludarabine and cyclophosphamide (FC) Limitations of use: • Initiate treatment with RITUXAN HYCELA only after patients have received at least one full d • RITUXAN HYCELA is not indicated for the treatment of non- conditions.
Sacituzumab govitecan-hziy/ TRODELVY Antibody-drug conjugate	Trop-2 Sacituzumab govitecan-hziy is a Trop-2-directed antibody-drug conjugate. Sacituzumab is a humanized antibody that recognizes Trop-2. The small molecule, SN-38, is a topoisomerase I inhibitor, which is covalently attached to the antibody by a linker. Pharmacology data suggest that sacituzumab govitecan-hziy binds to Trop-2-expressing cancer cells and is internalized with the subsequent release of SN-38 via hydrolysis of the linker. SN-38 interacts with topoisomerase I and prevents re-ligation of topoisomerase I-induced single strand breaks. The resulting DNA damage leads to apoptosis and cell death. Sacituzumab govitecan-hziy decreased tumor growth in mouse xenograft models of triple-negative breast cancer.	TRODELVY is a Trop-2-directed antibody and topoisomerase inhibitor conjugate indicated for the treatment of adult patients with metastatic triple-negative breast cancer (mTNBC) who have received at least two prior therapies for metastatic disease. This indication is approved under accelerated approval based on tumor response rate and duration of response. Continued approval for this indication may be contingent upon verification and description of clinical benefit in confirmatory trials

Sarilumab/ Kevzara/ fully human	IL-6 receptor	Adult patients with moderately to severely active rheumatoid arthritis who have had an inadequate response or intolerance to one or more disease-modifying antirheumatic drugs
Satralizumab-mwge/ Enspryng Humanized	Satralizumab is a humanized monoclonal antibody targeted against human IL-6 receptors. It binds to soluble and membrane-bound IL-6 receptors and prevents the signaling cascade, and subsequent pro-inflammatory effects, associated with its binding to endogenous IL-6.	Treatment of neuromyelitis optica spectrum disorder (NMOSD) in adult patients who are anti-aquaporin-4 (AQP4)
Secukinumab/ Cosentryx/ fully human	IL-17A (also known as IL-17)	Moderate to severe plaque psoriasis in adult patients who are candidates for systemic therapy or phototherapy.
Siltuximab/ Sylvant/ chimeric	IL-6	Multicentric Castleman's disease (MCD) who are human immunodeficiency virus (HIV) negative and human herpesvirus-8 (HHV-8) negative.
Tafasitamab-cxix/ MONJUVI	CD19	MONJUVI is a CD19-directed cytolytic antibody indicated in combination with lenalidomide for the treatment of adult patients with relapsed or refractory diffuse large B cell lymphoma (DLBCL) not otherwise specified, including DLBCL arising from low grade lymphoma, and who are not eligible for autologous stem cell transplant (ASCT). Tafasitamab-cxix is an Fc-modified monoclonal antibody that binds to CD19 antigen expressed on the surface of pre-B and mature B lymphocytes and on several B cell malignancies, including diffuse large B cell lymphoma (DLBCL). Upon binding to CD19, tafasitamab-cxix mediates B cell lysis through apoptosis and immune effector mechanisms, including antibody-dependent cellular cytotoxicity (ADCC) and antibody-dependent cellular phagocytosis (ADCP). This indication is approved under accelerated approval based on overall response rate. Continued approval for this indication may be contingent upon verification and description of clinical benefit in a confirmatory trial(s)
Teprotumumab-trbw/ TEPEZZA	IGFR Teprotumumab-trbw's mechanism of action in patients with	TEPEZZA is an insulin-like growth factor-1 receptor inhibitor indicated for the treatment of Thyroid Eye Disease

	Thyroid Eye Disease has not been fully characterized. Teprotumumab-trbw binds to IGF-1R and blocks its activation and signaling	
Tildrakizumab-asmn/Ilumya/ humanized	IL-23	Adults with moderate-to-severe plaque psoriasis who are candidates for systemic therapy or phototherapy
Tocilizumab/ Actrema/ humanized	IL-6 receptor	1. Rheumatoid arthritis (RA) • Adult patients with moderately to severely active rheumatoid arthritis who have had an inadequate response to one or more disease modifying anti-rheumatic drugs (DMARDs). 2.Giant cell arteritis (GCA) • Adult patients with giant cell arteritis. 3.Polyarticular juvenile idiopathic arthritis (PJIA) • Patients 2 years of age and older with active polyarticular juvenile idiopathic arthritis. 4.Systemic juvenile idiopathic arthritis (SJIA) • Patients 2 years of age and older with active systemic juvenile idiopathic arthritis. 5.Cytokine release syndrome (CRS) • Adults and pediatric patients 2 years of age and older with chimeric antigen receptor (CAR) T cell-induced severe or life-threatening cytokine release syndrome
Tratuzumab/ Herceptin/ humanized	HER2/neu	• HER2 overexpressing breast cancer •HER2-overexpressing metastatic gastric or gastroesophageal junction adenocarcinoma
Trastuzumab-dkst/Ogivri/ humanized biosimilar	HER2/neu	• HER2 overexpressing breast cancer •HER2-overexpressing metastatic gastric or gastroesophageal junction adenocarcinoma
Ustekinumab/ Stelara/ fully human	IL-12, IL-23	1. Adult patients with moderate to severe plaque psoriasis (Ps) who are candidates for phototherapy or systemic therapy. 2. Active psoriatic arthritis (PsA), alone or in combination with methotrexate. 3. Moderately to severely active Crohn's disease (CD) who have failed or were intolerant to treatment with immunomodulators or corticosteroids, but never failed a tumor necrosis factor (TNF) blocker or failed or were intolerant to treatment with one or more TNF blockers

		4. Adolescent patients (12 years or older) with moderate to severe plaque psoriasis, who are candidates for phototherapy or systemic therapy
Vedolizumab/ Entyvio/ humanized	Binds to the α4β7 integrin and blocks the interaction of α4β7 integrin with mucosal addressin cell adhesion molecule-1 (MAdCAM-1) and inhibits the migration of memory T lymphocytes across the endothelium into inflamed gastro-intestinal parenchymal tissue	1. Adult ulcerative colitis (UC) Adult patients with moderately to severely active UC who have had an inadequate response with, lost response to, or were intolerant to a tumor necrosis factor (TNF) blocker or immunomodulator; or had an inadequate response with, were intolerant to, or demonstrated dependence on corticosteroids • inducing and maintaining clinical response • inducing and maintaining clinical remission • improving endoscopic appearance of the mucosa 2. Achieving corticosteroid-free remission adult Crohn's disease (CD) • Adult patients with moderately to severely active CD who have had an inadequate response with, lost response to, or were intolerant to a TNF blocker or immunomodulator; or had an inadequate response with, were intolerant to, or demonstrated dependence on corticosteroids • achieving clinical response • achieving clinical remission • achieving corticosteroid-free remission

[a]Hidradenitis suppuriva is long term skin disease characterized by the occurrence of inflamed and swollen lumps

One other FDA-approved mab, tositumomab (Bexxar) (anti-CD20), was discontinued in 2014 due to lack of demand

[1]Burrill Bernard Crohn (1884 – 1983) was an American gastroenterologist

[2]Friedrich Sigmund Merkel (1845-1919) was a German anatomist and histopathologist

[3]Thomas Hodgkin (1798 – 1866) was a British physician

[4]Albert Sézary (1880 – 1956) was a French dermatologist and syphilogist

[5] Benjamin Castleman (1906 – 1982) was an American physician and pathologist

Examples of other biological therapeutics approved by the FDA for non- malignant diseases and malignant diseases

- Janus kinase inhibitors – eg, tofacitinib in Crohn's disease, ruxolitinib for steroid-refractory acute graft-versus-host disease
- Bruton's tyrosine kinase inhibitor – eg, ibrutinib for chronic graft-versus-host disease
- Other human tyrosine kinase inhibitors – eg, imatinib for systemic mastocytosis
- Angiogenesis inhibitors – eg, aflibercept for diabetic retinopathy
- Small interfering RNA-based drugs- eg, onasemnogene abeparvovec-xioi (Zolgensma) for familial amyloid polyneuropathy

Enzyme replacement treatments – eg, cerliponase alfa (Brineura) for Batten disease

Enzyme inhibitors – eg, lanadelumab-flyo (Takhzyro) for hereditary angioedema

Anti-sense drugs - eg, fomivirsen for cytomegalovirus retinitis, mipomersen for homozygous familial hypercholesterolemia, eteplirsen for Duchenne muscular dystrophy, nusinersen for spinal muscular atrophy

Cell therapies – Umbilical cord blood stem cells: FDA-approved for over 80 diseases, both non-malignant and malignant.

Gene-modified cell therapies

As of December 2020, the FDA had approved three different chimeric antigen receptor (CAR) T cell therapeutic agents for B cell acute lymphoblastic leukemia and aggressive non-Hodgkin lymphomas.

Gene therapies – eg, onasemnogene abeparvovec-xioi (Zolgensma) to treat spinal muscular atrophy type 1 has been approved for therapeutic use by the FDA. Voretigene neparvovec-rzyl (Luxturna) to treat congenital retinal dystrophy has also been approved by the FDA.

Hedgehog pathway inhibitors – eg sonidegib and vismodegib. These agents are chemically synthesised and FDA-approved for the treatment of advanced cutaneous squamous cell carcinoma or advanced basal cell carcinoma of the skin.

M-TOR inhibitors – eg sirolimus, temsirolimus and everolimus which inhibit the kinase activity of m-TOR, and which are used as immune suppressive agents

A list of small molecule protein kinase inhibitors approved by the USA FDA for therapeutic use (as of December 2020) is shown in Table 2.

Table 2. A list of small molecule protein kinase inhibitors approved by the USA FDA for therapeutic use.

Generic name/ trade name	Target and mechanism of action	FDA-approved indication/s
Abemaciclib/ Verzenio	Cyclin-dependent kinases 4 and 6 (CDK4 and CDK6). CDK4/6 inhibitor activity enforces G1 cell cycle arrest, and thus inhibits cellular proliferation	• In combination with an aromatase inhibitor as initial endocrine-based therapy for the treatment of postmenopausal women with hormone receptor (HR)-positive, human epidermal growth factor receptor 2 (HER2)-negative advanced or metastatic breast cancer. • in combination with fulvestrant for the treatment of women with hormone receptor (HR)-positive, human epidermal growth factor receptor 2 (HER2)-negative advanced or metastatic breast cancer with disease progression following endocrine therapy. • as monotherapy for the treatment of adult patients with HR positive, HER2-negative advanced or metastatic breast cancer with disease progression following endocrine therapy and prior chemotherapy in the metastatic setting.
Acalabrutinib/ Calquence	Bruton's tyrosine kinase[1]. (BTK). BTK is a signalling molecule of the B cell antigen receptor (BCR) and cytokine receptor pathways	1. Mantle cell lymphoma (MCL) who have received at least one prior therapy. This indication is approved under accelerated approval based on overall response rate. Continued approval for this indication may be contingent upon verification and description of clinical benefit in confirmatory trials 2. Chronic lymphocytic leukemia (CLL) or small lymphocytic lymphoma (SLL)
Afatinib/ Golotrif	ErbB (derived avian erythroblastosis oncogeneB). Signalling through the ErbB1/2/4 family of receptors promotes cell proliferation and opposes apoptosis. (ErbB is also known as, HER-2, HER-2/neu, HER2, NEU, CD340).	1. First-line treatment of patients with metastatic non-small cell lung cancer (NSCLC) whose tumors have non-resistant epidermal growth factor receptor (EGFR) mutations 2. Treatment of patients with metastatic, squamous NSCLC

	Afatinib covalently binds to the kinase domains of EGFR (ErbB1), HER2 (ErbB2), and HER4 (ErbB4) and irreversibly inhibits tyrosine kinase autophosphorylation, resulting in downregulation of ErbB signalling.	progressing after platinum-based chemotherapy
Alectinib/ Alecensa	ALK, RET. Alectinib is a tyrosine kinase inhibitor that targets ALK and RET. In non-clinical studies, alectinib inhibited ALK phosphorylation and ALK-mediated activation of the downstream signalling proteins STAT3 and AKT, and decreased tumor cell viability in multiple cell lines harboring ALK fusions, amplifications, or activating mutations.	Anaplastic lymphoma kinase (ALK)-positive metastatic non-small cell lung cancer (NSCLC)
Avapritinib/AYVAKIT	PDGFRA and PDGFRA D842 mutants Avapritinib is a tyrosine kinase inhibitor that targets PDGFRA and PDGFRA D842 mutants as well as multiple KIT exon 11, 11/17 and 17 mutants with half maximal inhibitory concentrations (IC50s) less than 25 nM. Certain mutations in PDGFRA and KIT can result in the autophosphorylation and constitutive activation of these receptors which can contribute to tumor cell proliferation. Other potential targets for avapritinib include wild type KIT, PDGFRB, and CSFR1. In in vitro cellular assays, avapritinib inhibited the autophosphorylation of KIT D816V and PDGFRA D842V, mutants associated with resistance to approved kinase inhibitors, with IC50 of 4 nM and 30 nM, respectively. Avapritinib also had anti-tumor activity in mice implanted with an imatinib-resistant patientderived xenograft model of human GIST with activating KIT exon 11/17 mutations.	AYVAKIT is a kinase inhibitor indicated for the treatment of adults with unresectable or metastatic gastrointestinal stromal tumor (GIST) harboring a platelet-derived growth factor receptor alpha (PDGFRA) exon 18 mutation, including PDGFRA D842V mutations.
Axitinib/Inlyta	Vascular endothelial growth factor receptors (VEGFR) 1/2/3. Axitinib has been shown to inhibit receptor tyrosine kinases including vascular endothelial growth factor receptors VEGFR-1, VEGFR-2, and VEGFR-3	Advanced renal cell carcinoma after failure of one prior systemic therapy

Baricitinib/ Olumiant	JAK1/2. Janus kinases phosphorylate activated cytokine receptors. These phosphorylated receptors in turn recruit STAT transcrip-tion factors which modulate gene transcription	Adult patients with moderately to severely active rheumatoid arthritis who have had an inadequate response to one or more TNF antagonist therapies
Binimetinib/ Mektovi	MEK1/2. MEK inhibitors inhibit the mitogen-activated protein kinase kinase enzymes MEK1and/or MEK2. They can be used to affect the MAPK/ERK pathway which is often overactive in some cancers	In combination with encorafenib, for the treatment of patients with unresectable or metastatic melanoma with a BRAF V600E or V600K mutation, as detected by an FDA-approved test.
Bosutinib/ Bosulif	BCR-ABL Bosutinib inhibits the BCR-ABL kinase that promotes CML	Treatment of adult patients with chronic, accelerated, or blast phase Ph+ chronic myelogenous leukemia (CML) with resistance or intolerance to prior therapy
Brigatinib/ Alunbrig	ALK. Brigatinib is a tyrosine kinase inhibitor with in vitro activity at clinically achievable concentrations against multiple kinases including ALK, ROS1, insulin-like growth factor-1 receptor (IGF-1R), and FLT-3 as well as EGFR deletion and point mutations. Brigatinib inhibited autophosphorylation of ALK and ALK-mediated phosphorylation of the downstream signalling proteins STAT3, AKT, ERK1/2, and S6 in in vitro and in vivo assays.	Patients with anaplastic lymphoma kinase (ALK)-positive metastatic non-small cell lung cancer (NSCLC) who have progressed on or are intolerant to crizotinib. This indication is approved under accelerated approval based on tumor response rate and duration of response. Continued approval for this indication may be contingent upon verification and description of clinical benefit in a confirmatory trial
Cabozantinib/ Cabometyx	RET, VEGFR2. Cabozantinib inhibits the tyrosine kinase activity of RET, MET, VEGFR-1, -2 and -3, KIT, TRKB, FLT-3, AXL, ROS1, TYRO3, MER, and TIE-2. These receptor tyrosine kinases are involved in both normal cellular function and pathologic processes such as oncogenesis, metastasis, tumor angiogenesis, drug resistance, and maintenance of the tumor microenvironment.	1.Patients with advanced renal cell carcinoma (RCC) 2. Patients with hepatocellular carcinoma (HCC) who have been previously treated with sorafenib
Cabozantinib/ Cometriq	RET, VEGFR2	Patients with progressive, metastatic medullary thyroid cancer (MTC)
Capmatinib/ TABRECTATM	MET Capmatinib is a kinase inhibitor that targets MET, including the mutant	TABRECTA is a kinase inhibitor indicated for the treatment of adult patients with metastatic non-small cell lung cancer (NSCLC) whose

	variant produced by exon 14 skipping. MET exon 14 skipping results in a protein with a missing regulatory domain that reduces its negative regulation leading to increased downstream MET signaling. Capmatinib inhibited cancer cell growth driven by a mutant MET variant lacking exon 14 at clinically achievable concentrations and demonstrated anti-tumor activity in murine tumor xenograft models derived from human lung tumors with either a mutation leading to MET exon 14 skipping or MET amplification. Capmatinib inhibited the phosphorylation of MET triggered by binding of hepatocyte growth factor or by MET amplification, as well as METmediated phosphorylation of downstream signaling proteins and proliferation and survival of MET-dependent cancer cells.	tumors have a mutation that leads to mesenchymal-epithelial transition (MET) exon 14 skipping as detected by an FDA-approved test. This indication is approved under accelerated approval based on overall response rate and duration of response. Continued approval for this indication may be contingent upon verification and description of clinical benefit in confirmatory trial(s).
Ceritinib/ Zykadia	ALK. Targets of ceritinib inhibition identified in either biochemical or cellular assays at clinically relevant concentrations include ALK, insulin-like growth factor 1 receptor (IGF-1R), insulin receptor (InsR), and ROS1. Among these, ceritinib is most active against ALK. Ceritinib inhibited autophosphorylation of ALK, ALK-mediated phosphorylation of the downstream signalling protein STAT3, and proliferation of ALK-dependent cancer cells in in vitro and in vivo assays.	Patients with metastatic non-small cell lung cancer (NSCLC) whose tumors are anaplastic lymphoma kinase (ALK)-positive
Cobimetinib/ Cotellic	MEK1/2. Cobimetinib is a reversible inhibitor of mitogen-activated protein kinase (MAPK)/extracellular signal regulated kinase 1 (MEK1) and MEK2. MEK proteins are upstream regulators of the extracellular signal related kinase (ERK) pathway, which promotes cellular proliferation. BRAF V600E and K mutations result in constitutive activation of the BRAF pathway which includes MEK1 and MEK2.	Unresectable or metastatic melanoma with a BRAF V600E or V600K mutation, in combination with vemurafenib
Crizotinib/ Xalkori	ALK, ROS1. Crizotinib is an inhibitor of receptor tyrosine kinases including ALK, Hepatocyte growth factor receptor (HGFR, c-Met), ROS1 (c-ros), and	Patients with metastatic non-small cell lung cancer (NSCLC) whose tumors are anaplastic lymphoma kinase (ALK) or ROS1-positive

	Recepteur d'Origine Nantais (RON). Translocations can affect the ALK gene resulting in the expression of oncogenic fusion proteins. The formation of ALK fusion proteins results in activation and dysregulation of the gene's expression and signalling which can contribute to increased cell proliferation and survival in tumors expressing these proteins.	
Dabrafenib/ Tafinlar	B-RAF. Dabrafenib is an inhibitor of some mutated forms of BRAF kinases with in vitro IC50 values of 0.65, 0.5, and 1.84 nM for BRAF V600E, BRAF V600K, and BRAF V600D enzymes, respectively. Dabrafenib also inhibits wild-type BRAF and CRAF kinases with IC50 values of 3.2 and 5.0 nM, respectively, and other kinases such as SIK1, NEK11, and LIMK1 at higher concentrations. Some mutations in the BRAF gene, including those that result in BRAF V600E, can result in constitutively activated BRAF kinases that may stimulate tumor cell growth.	TAFINLAR is a kinase inhibitor indicated as a single agent for the treatment of patients with unresectable or metastatic melanoma with BRAF V600E mutation as detected by an FDA-approved test. • TAFINLAR in combination with trametinib is indicated for the treatment of patients with unresectable or metastatic melanoma with BRAF V600E or V600K mutations as detected by an FDA-approved test. The use in combination is based on the demonstration of durable response rate. Improvement in disease-related symptoms or overall survival has not been demonstrated for TAFINLAR in combination with trametinib. Limitation of Use: TAFINLAR is not indicated for treatment of patients with wild-type BRAF melanoma.
Dacomitinib/ Vizimpro	EGFR. Dacomitinib is an irreversible inhibitor of the kinase activity of the human epidermal growth factor receptor (EGFR) family (EGFR/HER1, HER2, and HER4) and certain EGFR activating mutations (exon 19 deletion or the exon 21 L858R substitution mutation).	First-line treatment of patients with metastatic non-small cell lung cancer (NSCLC) with epidermal growth factor receptor (EGFR) exon 19 deletion or exon 21 L858R substitution mutations
Dasatinib/ Sprycell	BCR-ABL. Dasatinib, at nanomolar concentrations, inhibits the following kinases: BCR-ABL, SRC family (SRC, LCK, YES, FYN), c-KIT, EPHA2, and PDGFR-β. Based on modeling studies, dasatinib is	1. Newly diagnosed adults with Philadelphia chromosome-positive (Ph+) chronic myeloid leukemia (CML) in chronic phase. The trial is ongoing and further data will be required to determine long-term outcome. 2. Adults with chronic, accelerated, or myeloid or

	predicted to bind to multiple conformations of the ABL kinase.	lymphoid blast phase Ph+ CML with resistance or intolerance to prior therapy including imatinib. 3. Adults with Philadelphia chromosome-positive acute lymphoblastic leukemia (Ph+ ALL) with resistance or intolerance to prior therapy
Encorafenib/Braftovi	B-RAF. Encorafenib is a kinase inhibitor that targets BRAF V600E, as well as wild-type BRAF and CRAF in in vitro cell-free assays with IC50 values of 0.35, 0.47, and 0.3 nM, respectively. Mutations in the BRAF gene, such as BRAF V600E, can result in constitutively activated BRAF kinases that may stimulate tumor cell growth. Encorafenib was also able to bind to other kinases in vitro including JNK1, JNK2, JNK3, LIMK1, LIMK2, MEK4, and STK36 and substantially reduce ligand binding to these kinases at clinically achievable concentrations (≤ 0.9 μM).	BRAFTOVI is a kinase inhibitor indicated: • in combination with binimetinib, for the treatment of patients with unresectable or metastatic melanoma with a BRAF V600E or V600K mutation, as detected by an FDA-approved test. • in combination with cetuximab, for the treatment of adult patients with metastatic colorectal cancer (CRC) with a BRAF V600E mutation, as detected by an FDA-approved test, after prior therapy. Limitations of Use: BRAFTOVI is not indicated for treatment of patients with wild-type BRAF melanoma or wild-type BRAF CRC.
Entrectinib/ Rozlytrek	TRKA/B/C, ROS1, ALK. Entrectinib is an inhibitor of the tropomyosin receptor tyrosine kinases (TRK) TRKA, TRKB, and TRKC (encoded by the neurotrophic tyrosine receptor kinase [NTRK] genes NTRK1, NTRK2, and NTRK3, respectively), proto-oncogene tyrosine-protein kinase ROS1 (ROS1), and anaplastic lymphoma kinase (ALK). Fusion proteins that include TRK, ROS1, or ALK kinase domains can drive tumorigenic potential through hyperactivation of downstream signalling pathways leading to unconstrained cell proliferation.	• Adult patients with metastatic non-small cell lung cancer (NSCLC) whose tumors are ROS1-positive • Adult and pediatric patients 12 years of age and older with solid tumors that: o have a neurotrophic tyrosine receptor kinase (NTRK) gene fusion without a known acquired resistance mutation o are metastatic or where surgical resection is likely to result in severe morbidity o have progressed following treatment or have no satisfactory alternative therapy. This indication is approved under accelerated approval based on tumor response rate and durability of response. Continued approval for this indication may be contingent upon verification and

		description of clinical benefit in the confirmatory trials.
Erdafitinib/ Balversa	FGFR1/2/3/4. Erdafitinib is a kinase inhibitor that binds to and inhibits enzymatic activity of FGFR1, FGFR2, FGFR3 and FGFR4 based on in vitro data. Erdafitinib also binds to RET, CSF1R, PDGFRA, PDGFRB, FLT4, KIT, and VEGFR2. Erdafitinib inhibited FGFR phosphorylation and signalling and decreased cell viability in cell lines expressing FGFR genetic alterations, including point mutations, amplifications, and fusions. Erdafitinib demonstrated antitumor activity in FGFR-expressing cell lines and xenograft models derived from tumor types, including bladder cancer.	Treatment of adult patients with locally advanced or metastatic urothelial carcinoma that has • susceptible FGFR3 or FGFR2 genetic alterations and • progressed during or following at least one line of prior platinum-containing chemotherapy including within 12 months of neoadjuvant or adjuvant platinum-containing chemotherapy. This indication is approved under accelerated approval based on tumor response rate. Continued approval for this indication may be contingent upon verification and description of clinical benefit in confirmatory trials
Erlotinib/ Tarceva	EGFR. The mechanism of the clinical antitumor action of erlotinib is not fully characterized. Erlotinib inhibits the intracellular phosphorylation of tyrosine kinase associated with the epidermal growth factor receptor (EGFR). Specificity of inhibition with regard to other tyrosine kinase receptors has not been fully characterized. EGFR is expressed on the cell surface of normal cells and cancer cells.	1. Maintenance treatment of patients with locally advanced or metastatic non-small cell lung cancer (NSCLC) whose disease has not progressed after four cycles of platinum-based first-line chemotherapy. 2.Treatment of locally advanced or metastatic non-small cell lung cancer after failure of at least one prior chemotherapy regimen. 3.First-line treatment of patients with locally advanced, unresectable or metastatic pancreatic cancer, in combination with gemcitabine
Fedratinib/ Inrebic	JAK2, FLT3. Fedratinib is an oral kinase inhibitor with activity against wild type and mutationally activated Janus Associated Kinase 2 (JAK2) and FMS-like tyrosine kinase 3 (FLT3). Fedratinib is a JAK2-selective inhibitor with higher inhibitory activity for JAK2 over family members JAK1, JAK3 and TYK2. Abnormal activation of JAK2 is associated with myeloproliferative neoplasms (MPNs), including myelofibrosis and polycythemia vera	Treatment of adult patients with intermediate-2 or high-risk primary or secondary (post-polycythemia vera or post-essential thrombocythemia) myelofibrosis (MF)
Fostamatinib/	SYK.	Treatment of thrombocytopenia in adult patients with chronic immune thrombocytopenia (ITP)

Tavalisse	Fostamatinib is a tyrosine kinase inhibitor with demonstrated activity against spleen tyrosine kinase (SYK). The major metabolite of fostamatinib, R406, inhibits signal transduction of Fc-activating receptors and B cell receptor. The fostamatinib metabolite R406 reduces antibody-mediated destruction of platelets.	who have had an insufficient response to a previous treatment.
Gefitinib/ Iressa	EGFR. The epidermal growth factor receptor (EGFR) is expressed on the cell surface of both normal and cancer cells and plays a role in the processes of cell growth and proliferation. Some EGFR activating mutations (exon 19 deletion or exon 21 point mutation L858R) within NSCLC cells have been identified as contributing to the promotion of tumor cell growth, blocking of apoptosis, increasing the production of angiogenic factors and facilitating the processes of metastasis. Gefitinib reversibly inhibits the kinase activity of wild-type and certain activating mutations of EGFR, preventing autophosphorylation of tyrosine residues associated with the receptor, thereby inhibiting further downstream signalling and blocking EGFR-dependent proliferation. Gefitinib binding affinity for EGFR exon 19 deletion or exon 21 point mutation L858R mutations is higher than its affinity for the wild-type EGFR. Gefitinib also inhibits IGF and PDGF-mediated signalling at clinically relevant concentrations; inhibition of other tyrosine kinase receptors has not been fully characterized.	First-line treatment of patients with metastatic non-small cell lung cancer (NSCLC) whose tumors have epidermal growth factor receptor (EGFR) exon 19 deletions or exon 21 (L858R) substitution mutations. Limitation of use: the safety and efficacy of IRESSA have not been established in patients whose tumors have EGFR mutations other than exon 19 deletions or exon 21 (L858R) substitution mutations
Gilteritinib/ Xospata	Flt3. Gilteritinib is a small molecule that inhibits multiple receptor tyrosine kinases, including FMS-like tyrosine kinase 3 (FLT3). Gilteritinib demonstrated the ability to inhibit FLT3 receptor signalling and proliferation in cells exogenously expressing FLT3 including FLT3-ITD, tyrosine kinase domain mutations (TKD) FLT3-D835Y and FLT3-ITD-D835, and it induced apoptosis in leukemic cells expressing FLT3-ITD.	Treatment of adult patients who have relapsed or refractory acute myeloid leukemia (AML) with a FLT3 mutation

Ibrutinib/ Imbruvica	BTK. Ibrutinib is a small-molecule inhibitor of BTK. Ibrutinib forms a covalent bond with a cysteine residue in the BTK active site, leading to inhibition of BTK enzymatic activity. BTK is a signalling molecule of the B cell antigen receptor (BCR) and cytokine receptor pathways. BTK's role in signalling through the B cell surface receptors results in activation of pathways necessary for B cell trafficking, chemotaxis, and adhesion. Non-clinical studies show that ibrutinib inhibits B cell proliferation and survival in vivo as well as cell migration and substrate adhesion in vitro.	Treatment of adult patients with: 1. Mantle cell lymphoma (MCL) who have received at least one prior therapy. Accelerated approval was granted for this indication based on overall response rate. Continued approval for this indication may be contingent upon verification and description of clinical benefit in a confirmatory trial. 2. Chronic lymphocytic leukemia (CLL)/Small lymphocytic lymphoma (SLL) Chronic lymphocytic leukemia (CLL)/Small lymphocytic lymphoma (SLL) with 17p deletion 3. Waldenström's macroglobulinemia (WM) 4. Marginal zone lymphoma (MZL) who require systemic therapy and have received at least one prior anti-CD20-based therapy. Accelerated approval was granted for this indication based on overall response rate. Continued approval for this indication may be contingent upon verification and description of clinical benefit in a confirmatory trial. 5. Chronic graft-versus-host disease (cGVHD) after failure of one or more lines of systemic therapy
Imatinib/ Gleevec	Imatinib is tyrosine kinase specific for the TK domain in abl (the Abelson proto-oncogene), c-kit and PDGF-R (platelet-derived growth factor receptor.	1. Newly diagnosed adult and pediatric patients with Philadelphia chromosome positive chronic myeloid leukemia (Ph+ CML) in chronic phase 2. Patients with Philadelphia chromosome positive chronic myeloid leukemia (Ph+ CML) in blast crisis (BC), accelerated phase (AP), or in chronic phase (CP) after failure of interferon-alpha therapy 3. Adult patients with relapsed or refractory Philadelphia chromosome positive acute lymphoblastic leukemia (Ph+ ALL) 4. Pediatric patients with newly diagnosed Philadelphia chromosome positive acute

		lymphoblastic leukemia (Ph+ ALL) in combination with chemotherapy 5. Adult patients with myelodysplastic/myeloproliferative diseases (MDS/MPD) associated with platelet-derived growth factor receptor (PDGFR) gene re-arrangements 6. Adult patients with aggressive systemic mastocytosis (ASM) without the D816V c-Kit mutation or with c-Kit mutational status unknown 7. Adult patients with hypereosinophilic syndrome (HES) and/or chronic eosinophilic leukemia (CEL) who have the FIP1L1-PDGFR-α fusion kinase and for patients with HES and/or CEL who are FIP1L1 PDGFR-α fusion kinase negative or unknown 8. Adult patients with unresectable, recurrent and/or metastatic dermatofibrosarcoma protuberans (DFSP) 9. Patients with kit (CD117) positive unresectable and/or metastatic gastrointestinal stromal tumors (GIST) 10. Adjuvant treatment of adult patients following resection of kit (CD117) positive GIST
Lapatinib/ Tykerb	EGFR, ErbB2/HER2. Lapatinib is a 4-anilinoquinazoline kinase inhibitor of the intracellular tyrosine kinase domains of both Epidermal Growth Factor Receptor (EGFR [ErbB1]) and of Human Epidermal Receptor Type 2 (HER2 [ErbB2]). Lapatinib inhibits ErbB-driven tumor cell growth in vitro and in various animal models.	TYKERB, a kinase inhibitor, is indicated in combination with: • capecitabine, for the treatment of patients with advanced or metastatic breast cancer whose tumors overexpress HER2 and who have received prior therapy including an anthracycline, a taxane, and trastuzumab. • letrozole for the treatment of postmenopausal women with hormone receptor positive metastatic breast cancer that overexpresses the HER2 receptor for whom hormonal therapy is indicated. TYKERB in combination with an aromatase inhibitor has not been compared to a trastuzumab-

		containing chemotherapy regimen for the treatment of metastatic breast cancer
Larotrectinib/ Vitrakvi	TRKA/B/C. Larotrectinib is an inhibitor of the tropomyosin receptor kinases (TRK), TRKA, TRKB, and TRKC. In a broad panel of purified enzyme assays, larotrectinib inhibited TRKA, TRKB, and TRKC. TRKA, B, and C are encoded by the genes NTRK1, NTRK2, and NTRK3. Chromosomal rearrangements involving in-frame fusions of these genes with various partners can result in constitutively-activated chimeric TRK fusion proteins that can act as an oncogenic driver, promoting cell proliferation and survival in tumor cell lines.	Treatment of adult and pediatric patients with solid tumors that • have a neurotrophic receptor tyrosine kinase (NTRK) gene fusion without a known acquired resistance mutation • are metastatic or where surgical resection is likely to result in severe morbidity, and • have no satisfactory alternative treatments or that have progressed following treatment. This indication is approved under accelerated approval based on overall response rate and duration of response. Continued approval for this indication may be contingent upon verification and description of clinical benefit in confirmatory trials.
Lenvatinib/ Lenvima	VEGFR, FGFR, RET, PDGFR, KIT. Lenvatinib is a kinase inhibitor that inhibits the kinase activities of vascular endothelial growth factor (VEGF) receptors VEGFR1 (FLT1), VEGFR2 (KDR), and VEGFR3 (FLT4). Lenvatinib inhibits other kinases that have been implicated in pathogenic angiogenesis, tumor growth, and cancer progression in addition to their normal cellular functions, including fibroblast growth factor (FGF) receptors FGFR1, 2, 3, and 4; platelet derived growth factor receptor alpha (PDGFRα), KIT, and RET. Lenvatinib also exhibited antiproliferative activity in hepatocellular carcinoma cell lines dependent on activated FGFR signalling with a concurrent inhibition of FGF-receptor substrate 2α (FRS2α) phosphorylation. The combination of lenvatinib and everolimus showed increased antiangiogenic and antitumor activity as demonstrated by decreases in human endothelial cell proliferation, tube formation, and VEGF signalling in vitro, and by decreases in tumor volume in mouse xenograft models of human renal cell cancer that were	Treatment of patients with 1. Locally recurrent or metastatic, progressive, radioactive iodine-refractory differentiated thyroid cancer (DTC). 2. In combination with everolimus, for the treatment of patients with advanced renal cell carcinoma (RCC) following one prior antiangiogenic therapy. 3. For the first-line treatment of patients with unresectable hepatocellular carcinoma (HCC)

	greater than those with either drug alone.	
Lonafarnib	Lonafarnib inhibits farnesyltransferase to prevent farnesylation and subsequent accumulation of progerin and progerin-like proteins in the inner nuclear membrane.	ZOKINVY is a farnesyltransferase inhibitor indicated in patients 12 months of age and older with a body surface area of 0.39 m^2 and above • To reduce risk of mortality in Hutchinson-Gilford Progeria Syndrome • For treatment of processing-deficient Progeroid Laminopathies with either: o Heterozygous LMNA mutation with progerin-like protein accumulation o Homozygous or compound heterozygous ZMPSTE24 mutations
Lorlatinib/ Lorbrena	ALK, ROS1 and others. Lorlatinib is a kinase inhibitor with in vitro activity against ALK and ROS1 as well as TYK1, FER, FPS, TRKA, TRKB, TRKC, FAK, FAK2, and ACK. Lorlatinib demonstrated in vitro activity against multiple mutant forms of the ALK enzyme, including some mutations detected in tumors at the time of disease progression on crizotinib and other ALK inhibitors.	Treatment of patients with anaplastic lymphoma kinase (ALK)-positive metastatic non-small cell lung cancer (NSCLC) whose disease has progressed on • crizotinib and at least one other ALK inhibitor for metastatic disease • or on alectinib as the first ALK inhibitor therapy for metastatic disease • or on ceritinib as the first ALK inhibitor therapy for metastatic disease. This indication is approved under accelerated approval based on tumor response rate and duration of response. Continued approval for this indication may be contingent upon verification and description of clinical benefit in a confirmatory trial.
Midostaurin/ Rydapt	Flt3. Midostaurin is a small molecule that inhibits multiple receptor tyrosine kinases. In vitro biochemical or cellular assays have shown that midostaurin or its major human active metabolites CGP62221 and CGP52421 inhibit the activity of wild type FLT3, FLT3 mutant kinases (ITD and TKD), KIT (wild type and D816V	Treatment of adult patients with: newly diagnosed acute myeloid leukemia (AML) that is FLT3 mutation-positive in combination with standard cytarabine and daunorubicin induction and cytarabine consolidation. Limitations of use: RYDAPT is not indicated as a single-agent induction therapy for the

	mutant), PDGFRα/β, VEGFR2, as well as members of the serine/threonine kinase PKC (protein kinase C) family.	treatment of patients with AML, aggressive systemic mastocytosis (ASM), systemic mastocytosis with associated hematological neoplasm (SM-AHN), or mast cell leukemia (MCL).
Neratinib/ Nerlynx	ErbB2/HER2. A kinase inhibitor that irreversibly binds to Epidermal Growth Factor Receptor (EGFR), Human Epidermal Growth Factor Receptor 2 (HER2), and HER4. In vitro, neratinib reduces EGFR and HER2 autophosphorylation, downstream MAPK and AKT signalling pathways, and showed antitumor activity in EGFR and/or HER2 expressing carcinoma cell lines. Neratinib human metabolites M3, M6, M7 and M11 inhibited the activity of EGFR, HER2 and HER4 in vitro. In vivo, oral administration of neratinib inhibited tumor growth in mouse xenograft models with tumor cell lines expressing HER2 and EGFR.	NERLYNX is a kinase inhibitor indicated: • As a single agent, for the extended adjuvant treatment of adult patients with early stage HER2-positive breast cancer, to follow adjuvant trastuzumabbased therapy. • In combination with capecitabine, for the treatment of adult patients with advanced or metastatic HER2-positive breast cancer who have received two or more prior anti-HER2 based regimens in the metastatic setting.
Netarsudil/ Rhopressa	ROCK1/2 (Rho associated coiled-coil containing protein kinase 1) Netarsudil is a rho kinase inhibitor, which is believed to reduce intra-ocular pressure (IOP) by increasing the outflow of aqueous humor through the trabecular meshwork route. The exact mechanism is unknown.	RHOPRESSA® (netarsudil ophthalmic solution) 0.02% is a Rho kinase inhibitor indicated for the reduction of elevated intraocular pressure in patients with open-angle glaucoma or ocular hypertension
Nilotinib/ Tasigna	BCR-ABL. Nilotinib is an inhibitor of the BCR-ABL kinase.	1. Treatment of newly diagnosed adult patients with Philadelphia chromosome positive chronic myeloid leukemia (Ph+ CML) in chronic phase. 2. Treatment of chronic phase (CP) and accelerated phase (AP) Ph+ CML in adult patients resistant to or intolerant to prior therapy that included imatinib.
Nintedanib/ Vargatef	Multiple kinases. Nintedanib is a small molecule that inhibits multiple receptor tyrosine kinases (RTKs) and non-receptor tyrosine kinases (nRTKs). Nintedanib inhibits the following RTKs: platelet-derived growth factor receptor (PDGFR) α and β, fibroblast growth factor receptor (FGFR) 1-3, vascular endothelial growth factor receptor	The treatment of idiopathic pulmonary fibrosis (IPF).

	(VEGFR) 1-3, and Fms-like tyrosine kinase-3 (FLT3). Among them, FGFR, PDGFR, and VEGFR have been implicated in IPF pathogenesis. Nintedanib binds competitively to the adenosine triphosphate (ATP) binding pocket of these receptors and blocks the intracellular signalling which is crucial for the proliferation, migration, and transformation of fibroblasts representing essential mechanisms of the IPF pathology.	
Osimertinib/ Tagrisso	EGFR Osimertinib is a kinase inhibitor of the epidermal growth factor receptor (EGFR), which binds irreversibly to certain mutant forms of EGFR (T790M, L858R, and exon 19 deletion) at approximately 9- fold lower concentrations than wild-type. In vitro, osimertinib also inhibited the activity of HER2, HER3, HER4, ACK1, and BLK at clinically relevant concentrations. In cultured cells and animal tumor implantation models, osimertinib exhibited anti-tumor activity against NSCLC lines harboring EGFR-mutations (T790M/L858R, L858R, T790M/exon 19 deletion, and exon 19 deletion) and, to a lesser extent, wild-type EGFR amplifications	1. The first-line treatment of patients with metastatic NSCLC whose tumors have epidermal growth factor receptor (EGFR) exon 19 deletions or exon 21 L858R mutations 2. The treatment of patients with metastatic EGFR T790M mutation-positive NSCLC whose disease has progressed on or after EGFR TKI therapy
Palbociclib/ Ibrance	CDK4/6	IBRANCE is a kinase inhibitor indicated for the treatment of adult patients with hormone receptor (HR)-positive, human epidermal growth factor receptor 2 (HER2)-negative advanced or metastatic breast cancer in combination with: • an aromatase inhibitor as initial endocrine-based therapy in postmenopausal women or in men; or • fulvestrant in patients with disease progression following endocrine therapy.
Pazopanib/ Votrient	VEGFR1/2/3 Pazopanib is a multi-tyrosine kinase inhibitor of vascular endothelial growth factor receptor (VEGFR)-1, VEGFR-2, VEGFR-3, platelet-derived growth factor receptor (PDGFR)-α and -β, fibroblast growth factor receptor (FGFR) -1 and -3, cytokine	The treatment of patients with: 1. Advanced renal cell carcinoma 2. Advanced soft tissue sarcoma who have received prior chemotherapy. Limitations of use: the efficacy of VOTRIENT for the treatment of

	receptor (Kit), interleukin-2, receptor inducible T cell kinase (Itk), leukocyte-specific protein tyrosine kinase (Lck), and transmembrane glycoprotein receptor tyrosine kinase (c-fms). In vitro, pazopanib inhibited ligand-induced autophosphorylation of VEGFR-2, Kit and PDGFR-β receptors. In vivo, pazopanib inhibited VEGF-induced VEGFR-2 phosphorylation in mouse lungs, angiogenesis in a mouse model, and the growth of some human tumor xenografts in mice.	patients with adipocytic soft tissue sarcoma or gastrointestinal stromal tumors has not been demonstrated.
Pemigatinib/ PEMAZYRE™	FGFR2 Pemigatinib is a small molecule kinase inhibitor that targets FGFR1, 2 and 3 with IC50 values of less than 2 nM. Pemigatinib also inhibited FGFR4 in vitro at a concentration approximately 100 times higher than those that inhibit FGFR1, 2, and 3. Pemigatinib inhibited FGFR1-3 phosphorylation and signaling and decreased cell viability in cancer cell lines with activating FGFR amplifications and fusions that resulted in constitutive activation of FGFR signaling. Constitutive FGFR signaling can support the proliferation and survival of malignant cells. Pemigatinib exhibited anti-tumor activity in mouse xenograft models of human tumors with FGFR1, FGFR2, or FGFR3 alterations resulting in constitutive FGFR activation including a patient-derived xenograft model of cholangiocarcinoma that expressed an oncogenic FGFR2 Transformer-2 beta homolog (TRA2b) fusion protein.	PEMAZYRE is a kinase inhibitor indicated for the treatment of adults with previously treated, unresectable locally advanced or metastatic cholangiocarcinoma with a fibroblast growth factor receptor 2 (FGFR2) fusion or other rearrangement as detected by an FDA-approved test. This indication is approved under accelerated approval based on overall response rate and duration of response. Continued approval for this indication may be contingent upon verification and description of clinical benefit in a confirmatory trial(s).
Pexidartinib/ Turalio	Multiple kinases. Pexidartinib is a small molecule tyrosine kinase inhibitor that targets colony stimulating factor 1 receptor (CSF1R), KIT proto-oncogene receptor tyrosine kinase (KIT), and FMS-like tyrosine kinase 3 (FLT3) harboring an internal tandem duplication (ITD) mutation. Overexpression of the CSF1R ligand promotes cell proliferation and accumulation in the synovium. In vitro, pexidartinib inhibited proliferation of cell lines dependent on CSF1R and ligand-induced autophosphorylation of CSF1R.	The treatment of adult patients with symptomatic tenosynovial giant cell tumor (TGCT) associated with severe morbidity or functional limitations and not amenable to improvement with surgery.

	Pexidartinib also inhibited the proliferation of a CSF1R dependent cell line in vivo.	
Ponatinib/ Iclusig	ABL Ponatinib inhibited the in vitro tyrosine kinase activity of ABL and T315I mutant ABL with IC50 concentrations of 0.4 and 2.0 nM, respectively. Ponatinib inhibited the in vitro activity of additional kinases with IC50 concentrations between 0.1 and 20 nM, including members of the VEGFR, PDGFR, FGFR, EPH receptors and SRC families of kinases, and KIT, RET, TIE2, and FLT3. Ponatinib inhibited the in vitro viability of cells expressing native or mutant BCR-ABL, including T315I. In mice, treatment with ponatinib reduced the size of tumors expressing native or T315I mutant BCR-ABL when compared to controls.	Iclusig is a kinase inhibitor indicated for the: 1. Treatment of adult patients with chronic phase, accelerated phase, or blast phase chronic myeloid leukemia (CML) or Ph+ ALL for whom no other tyrosine kinase inhibitor (TKI) therapy is indicated. 2. Treatment of adult patients with T315I-positive CML (chronic phase, accelerated phase, or blast phase) or T315I-positive Philadelphia chromosome positive acute lymphoblastic leukemia (Ph+ ALL)
Pralsetinib/Gavreto	Kinase inhibitor of wild-type RET and oncogenic RET fusions and mutations.	For the treatment of adult patients with metastatic RET fusion-positive non-small cell lung cancer (NSCLC) as detected by an FDA approved test
Regorafenib/ Tafinlar	VEGFR1/2/3 Regorafenib is a small molecule inhibitor of multiple membrane-bound and intracellular kinases involved in normal cellular functions and in pathologic processes such as oncogenesis, tumor angiogenesis, and maintenance of the tumor microenvironment. In in vitro biochemical or cellular assays, regorafenib or its major human active metabolites M-2 and M-5 inhibited the activity of RET, VEGFR1, VEGFR2, VEGFR3, KIT, PDGFR-alpha, PDGFR-beta, FGFR1, FGFR2, TIE2, DDR2, Trk2A, Eph2A, RAF-1, BRAF, BRAFV600E , SAPK2, PTK5, and Abl at concentrations of regorafenib that have been achieved clinically. In in vivo models, regorafenib demonstrated anti-angiogenic activity in a rat tumor model, and inhibition of tumor growth as well as anti-metastatic activity in several mouse xenograft models including some for human colorectal carcinoma.	Metastatic colorectal cancer (CRC) who have been previously treated with fluoropyrimidine-, oxaliplatin- and irinotecan-based chemotherapy, an anti-VEGF therapy, and, if KRAS wild type, an anti-EGFR therapy

Ribociclib/ Kisqali	CDK4/6 Ribociclib is an inhibitor of cyclin-dependent kinase (CDK) 4 and 6. These kinases are activated upon binding to Dcyclins and play a crucial role in signalling pathways which lead to cell cycle progression and cellular proliferation. The cyclin D-CDK4/6 complex regulates cell cycle progression through phosphorylation of the retinoblastoma protein (pRb). In vitro, ribociclib decreased pRb phosphorylation leading to arrest in the G1 phase of the cell cycle and reduced cell proliferation in non-Hodgkin's lymphoma cell lines. In vivo, treatment with single agent ribociclib in a rat xenograft model with human tumor cells led to decreased tumor volumes, which correlated with inhibition of pRb phosphorylation.	IBRANCE is a kinase inhibitor indicated for the treatment of adult patients with hormone receptor (HR)-positive, human epidermal growth factor receptor 2 (HER2)-negative advanced or metastatic breast cancer in combination with: • an aromatase inhibitor as initial endocrine-based therapy in postmenopausal women or in men; or • fulvestrant in patients with disease progression following endocrine therapy
Ripretinib/ QINLOCK™	KIT, PDGFRA	QINLOCK is a kinase inhibitor indicated for the treatment of adult patients with advanced gastrointestinal stromal tumor (GIST) who have received prior treatment with 3 or more kinase inhibitors, including imatinib. Ripretinib is a tyrosine kinase inhibitor that inhibits KIT proto-oncogene receptor tyrosine kinase (KIT) and platelet derived growth factor receptor A (PDGFRA) kinase, including wild type, primary, and secondary mutations. Ripretinib also inhibits other kinases in vitro, such as PDGFRB, TIE2, VEGFR2, and BRAF.
Ruxolitinib/ Jakafi	JAK1/2/3,Tyk Ruxolitinib, a kinase inhibitor, inhibits Janus Associated Kinases (JAKs) JAK1 and JAK2 which mediate the signalling of a number of cytokines and growth factors that are important for hematopoiesis and immune function. JAK signalling involves recruitment of STATs (signal transducers and activators of transcription) to cytokine receptors, activation and subsequent localization of STATs to the nucleus leading to modulation of gene expression. Myelofibrosis (MF) is a	Jakafi is a kinase inhibitor indicated for treatment of patients with intermediate or high-risk myelofibrosis, including primary myelofibrosis, post-polycythemia vera myelofibrosis and post-essential thrombocythemia myelofibrosis

	myeloproliferative neoplasm (MPN) known to be associated with dysregulated JAK1 and JAK2 signalling. In a mouse model of JAK2V617F-positive MPN, oral administration of ruxolitinib prevented splenomegaly, preferentially decreased JAK2V617F mutant cells in the spleen and decreased circulating inflammatory cytokines (eg, TNF-α, IL-6).	
Selpercatinib/ RETEVMO	RET Selpercatinib is a kinase inhibitor. Selpercatinib inhibited wild-type RET and multiple mutated RET isoforms as well as VEGFR1 and VEGFR3 with IC50 values ranging from 0.92 nM to 67.8 nM. In other enzyme assays, selpercatinib also inhibited FGFR 1, 2, and 3 at higher concentrations that were still clinically achievable. In cellular assays, selpercatinib inhibited RET at approximately 60-fold lower concentrations than FGFR1 and 2 and approximately 8-fold lower concentration than VEGFR3. Certain point mutations in RET or chromosomal rearrangements involving in-frame fusions of RET with various partners can result in constitutively activated chimeric RET fusion proteins that can act as oncogenic drivers by promoting cell proliferation of tumor cell lines. In in vitro and in vivo tumor models, selpercatinib demonstrated anti-tumor activity in cells harboring constitutive activation of RET protein resulting from gene fusions and mutations, including CCDC6-RET, KIF5B-RET, RET V804M, and RET M918T. In addition, selpercatinib showed anti-tumor activity in mice intracranially implanted with a patient-derived RET fusion positive tumor.	RETEVMO is a kinase inhibitor indicated for the treatment of: • Adult patients with metastatic RET fusion-positive non-small cell lung cancer (NSCLC)1 • Adult and pediatric patients 12 years of age and older with advanced or metastatic RET-mutant medullary thyroid cancer (MTC) who require systemic therapy • Adult and pediatric patients 12 years of age and older with advanced or metastatic RET fusion-positive thyroid cancer who require systemic therapy and who are radioactive iodine-refractory (if radioactive iodine is appropriate). 1 This indication is approved under accelerated approval based on overall response rate and duration of response. Continued approval for this indication may be contingent upon verification and description of clinical benefit in confirmatory Selpercatinib is a kinase inhibitor. Selpercatinib inhibited wild-type RET and multiple mutated RET isoforms as well as VEGFR1 and VEGFR3 with IC50 values ranging from 0.92 nM to 67.8 nM. In other enzyme assays, selpercatinib also inhibited FGFR 1, 2, and 3 at higher concentrations that were still clinically achievable. In cellular assays, selpercatinib inhibited RET at approximately 60-fold lower concentrations than FGFR1 and 2 and approximately 8-fold lower concentration than VEGFR3. Certain point mutations in RET or chromosomal rearrangements involving in-frame fusions of RET with various partners can result in

		constitutively activated chimeric RET fusion proteins that can act as oncogenic drivers by promoting cell proliferation of tumor cell lines. In in vitro and in vivo tumor models, selpercatinib demonstrated anti-tumor activity in cells harboring constitutive activation of RET protein resulting from gene fusions and mutations, including CCDC6-RET, KIF5B-RET, RET V804M, and RET M918T. In addition, selpercatinib showed Reference ID: 4605720 anti-tumor activity in mice intracranially implanted with a patient-derived RET fusion positive tumor trial(s).
Selumetinib/ KOSELUGO	MEK1/2 Selumetinib is an inhibitor of mitogen-activated protein kinase kinases 1 and 2 (MEK1/2). MEK1/2 proteins are upstream regulators of the extracellular signal-related kinase (ERK) pathway. Both MEK and ERK are critical components of the RAS-regulated RAF-MEK-ERK pathway, which is often activated in different types of cancers. In genetically modified mouse models of NF1 that generate neurofibromas that recapitulate the genotype and phenotype of human NF1, oral dosing of selumetinib inhibited ERK phosphorylation, and reduced neurofibroma numbers, volume, and proliferation.	KOSELUGO is a kinase inhibitor indicated for the treatment of pediatric patients 2 years of age and older with neurofibromatosis type 1 (NF1) who have symptomatic, inoperable plexiform neurofibromas (PN).
Sorafenib/ Nexavar	VEGFR1/2/3 Sorafenib has been shown to inhibit multiple intracellular (c-CRAF, BRAF and mutant BRAF) and cell surface kinases (KIT, FLT- 3, RET, RET/PTC, VEGFR-1, VEGFR- 2, VEGFR- 3, and PDGFR-ß). Several of these kinases are thought to be involved in tumor cell signalling, angiogenesis and apoptosis. Sorafenib inhibited tumor growth of HCC, RCC, and DTC human tumor xenografts in immunocompromised mice. Reductions in tumor angiogenesis were seen in models of HCC and RCC upon sorafenib treatment, and increases in tumor apoptosis were observed in models of HCC, RCC, and DTC.	Treatment of 1.Unresectable hepatocellular carcinoma (HCC) 2. Advanced renal cell carcinoma (RCC) 3. Locally recurrent or metastatic, progressive, differentiated thyroid carcinoma (DTC) refractory to radioactive iodine treatment

Sunitinib/ Sutent	Multiple kinases. Sunitinib is a small molecule that inhibits multiple receptor tyrosine kinases (RTKs), some of which are implicated in tumor growth, pathologic angiogenesis, and metastatic progression of cancer. Sunitinib was evaluated for its inhibitory activity against a variety of kinases (>80 kinases) and was identified as an inhibitor of platelet-derived growth factor receptors (PDGFRα and PDGFRβ), vascular endothelial growth factor receptors (VEGFR1, VEGFR2 and VEGFR3), stem cell factor receptor (KIT), Fms-like tyrosine kinase-3 (FLT3), colony stimulating factor receptor Type 1 (CSF-1R), and the glial cell-line derived neurotrophic factor receptor (RET). Sunitinib inhibited the phosphorylation of multiple RTKs (PDGFRβ, VEGFR2, KIT) in tumor xenografts expressing RTK targets in vivo and demonstrated inhibition of tumor growth or tumor regression and/or inhibited metastases in some experimental models of cancer. Sunitinib demonstrated the ability to inhibit growth of tumor cells expressing dysregulated target RTKs (PDGFR, RET, or KIT) in vitro and to inhibit PDGFRβ- and VEGFR2-dependent tumor angiogenesis in vivo.	The treatment of: 1. Gastrointestinal stromal tumor (GIST) after disease progression on or intolerance to imatinib mesylate. 2. Advanced renal cell carcinoma (RCC). 3. Progressive, well-differentiated pancreatic neuroendocrine tumors (pNET) in patients with unresectable locally advanced or metastatic disease
Tofacitinib/ Xeljanz/ Xeljanz XR	JAK Tofacitinib is a Janus kinase (JAK) inhibitor. JAKs are intracellular enzymes which transmit signals arising from cytokine or growth factor-receptor interactions on the cellular membrane to influence cellular processes of hematopoiesis and immune cell function. Within the signalling pathway, JAKs phosphorylate and activate Signal Transducers and Activators of Transcription (STATs) which modulate intracellular activity including gene expression. Tofacitinib modulates the signalling pathway at the point of JAKs, preventing the phosphorylation and activation of 26 Reference ID: 4467787 STATs. JAK enzymes transmit cytokine signalling through pairing of JAKs (e.g., JAK1/JAK3, JAK1/JAK2, JAK1/TyK2, JAK2	1. Rheumatoid arthritis: XELJANZ/XELJANZ XR is indicated for the treatment of adult patients with moderately to severely active rheumatoid arthritis who have had an inadequate response or intolerance to methotrexate. It may be used as monotherapy or in combination with methotrexate or other non-biologic disease-modifying antrheumatic drugs (DMARDs). ○ Limitations of use: use of XELJANZ/XELJANZ XR in combination with biologic DMARDs or potent immunosuppressants such as azathioprine and cyclosporine is not recommended. 2. Psoriatic arthritis: XELJANZ/XELJANZ XR is

	/JAK2). Tofacitinib inhibited the in vitro activities of JAK1/JAK2, JAK1/JAK3, and JAK2/JAK2 combinations with IC50 of 406, 56, and 1377 nM, respectively. However, the relevance of specific JAK combinations to therapeutic effectiveness is not known.	indicated for the treatment of adult patients with active psoriatic arthritis who have had an inadequate response or intolerance to methotrexate or other disease-modifying anti-rheumatic drugs (DMARDs). ○ Limitations of use: use of XELJANZ/XELJANZ XR in combination with biologic DMARDs or potent immunosuppressants such as azathioprine and cyclosporine is not recommended. 3. Ulcerative colitis: XELJANZ is indicated for the treatment of adult patients with moderately to severely active ulcerative colitis (UC), who have had an inadequate response or who are intolerant to TNF blockers. ○ Limitations of use: use of XELJANZ in combination with biological therapies for UC or with potent immunosuppressants such as azathioprine and cyclosporine is not recommended.
Trametinib/ Mekinist	MEK1/2 Trametinib is a reversible inhibitor of mitogen-activated extracellular signal-regulated kinase 1 (MEK1) and MEK2 activation and of MEK1 and MEK2 kinase activity. MEK proteins are upstream regulators of the extracellular signal-related kinase (ERK) pathway, which promotes cellular proliferation. BRAF V600E mutations result in constitutive activation of the BRAF pathway which includes MEK1 and MEK2. Trametinib inhibits cell growth of various BRAF V600 mutation-positive tumors in vitro and in vivo. Trametinib and dabrafenib target two different kinases in the RAS/RAF/MEK/ERK pathway. Use of trametinib and dabrafenib in combination resulted in greater growth inhibition of BRAF V600 mutation-positive tumor cell lines in vitro and prolonged inhibition of tumor growth in BRAF V600 mutation positive tumor xenografts compared with either drug alone.	MEKINIST is a kinase inhibitor indicated as a single agent for the treatment of patients with unresectable or metastatic melanoma with BRAF V600E or V600K mutations as detected by an FDA-approved test. MEKINIST is indicated, in combination with dabrafenib, for: • the treatment of patients with unresectable or metastatic melanoma with BRAF V600E or V600K mutations as detected by an FDA-approved test. • the adjuvant treatment of patients with melanoma with BRAF V600E or V600K mutations, as detected by an FDA-approved test, and involvement of lymph node(s), following complete resection. • the treatment of patients with metastatic non-small cell lung cancer (NSCLC) with BRAF V600E mutation as detected by an FDA-approved test.

		Limitation of Use: MEKINIST is not indicated for treatment of patients with melanoma who have progressed on prior BRAF-inhibitor therapy
Tucatinib/TUKYSA	HER2 Tucatinib is a tyrosine kinase inhibitor of HER2. In vitro, tucatinib inhibits phosphorylation of HER2 and HER3, resulting in inhibition of downstream MAPK and AKT signaling and cell proliferation, and showed antitumor activity in HER2 expressing tumor cells. In vivo, tucatinib inhibited the growth of HER2 expressing tumors. The combination of tucatinib and trastuzumab showed increased anti-tumor activity in vitro and in vivo compared to either drug alone.	TUKYSA is a kinase inhibitor indicated in combination with trastuzumab and capecitabine for treatment of adult patients with advanced unresectable or metastatic HER2-positive breast cancer, including patients with brain metastases, who have received one or more prior anti-HER2-based regimens in the metastatic setting
Vemurafenib/ Zalora	B-Raf Vemurafenib is a low molecular weight, orally available inhibitor of some mutated forms of BRAF serine-threonine kinase, including BRAF V600E. Vemurafenib also inhibits other kinases in vitro such as CRAF, ARAF, wild-type BRAF, SRMS, ACK1, MAP4K5, and FGR at similar concentrations. Some mutations in the BRAF gene including V600E result in constitutively activated BRAF proteins, which can cause cell proliferation in the absence of growth factors that would normally be required for proliferation. Vemurafenib has anti-tumor effects in cellular and animal models of melanoma with mutated BRAF V600E.	ZELBORAF® is a kinase inhibitor indicated for the treatment of patients with unresectable or metastatic melanoma with BRAF V600E mutation as detected by an FDA-approved test. Limitation of Use: ZELBORAF is not indicated for treatment of patients with wild-type BRAF melanoma.
Upadacitinib/Rinvaq	Janus kinase inhibitor	The treatment of adults with moderately to severely active rheumatoid arthritis who have had an inadequate response or intolerance to methotrexate. Limitation of use: use of RINVOQ in combination with other JAK inhibitors, biologic DMARDs, or with potent immunosuppressants such as azathioprine and cyclosporine is not recommended

To this list can now be added the CAR T cell therapies approved by the USA FDA for therapeutic use (Table 3).

Table 3. FDA-approved CAR T cell therapies.

Generic name	**Brand name**	**Target antigen**	**Targeted disease**	**Patient population**
Tisagenlecleucel	Kymriah	CD19	B cell acute lymphoblastic leukemia (ALL); B cell non-Hodgkin lymphoma (NHL)	Children and young adults with refractory or relapsed (r/r) B cell ALL Adults with r/y B cell NHL
Axicabtagene ciloleucel	Yescarta	CD19	B cell NHL Follicular lymphoma	Adults with r/r B cell NHL Adults with r/r follicular NHL
Brexucabtagene autoleucel	Tecartus	CD19	Mantle cell lymphoma (MCL) B cell ALL	Adults with r/r MCL Adults with r/r B cell ALL

Lisocabtagene maraleucel	Breyanzi	CD19	B cell NHL	Adults with r/ry B cell NHL
Idecabtagene vicleucel	Abecma	B cell maturation antigen (BCMA)	Multiple myeloma (MM)	Adults with r/r MM
Ciltacabtagene autoleucel	Carvikti	BCMA	MM	Adults with r/r MM

[1]Ogden Carr Bruton (1908 - 2003) was an American pediatrician

Summary of treatments derived from of the biological discoveries in the last 70 years

94 monoclonal antibodies (including biosimilars) and 59 small molecule protein kinase inhibitors are now FDA-approved for therapeutic purposes. Additional classes of therapeutics include new cellular therapies including gene-modified cellular therapies and gene therapies.

All these agents will be described in detail in each book on diseases for which they have been approved. This book deals only with the use of **CAR T cell therapies.** It is one in a series of books on the impact of targeted biological and specifically designed therapeutic agents across the whole field of medicine in a series called Medicine 2020.

3. The biology of normal human cells

To fully understand how these new therapeutic agents work it is useful to understand how cells work – in particular what signalling pathways they use. Normal cells and cells in tissues affected by non- diseases use signalling pathways often different from those used by cells.

All human cells are derived from a single totipotent stem cell which is produced by the fusion of a single sperm with a single ovum. This totipotent stem cell has all the genes on its chromosomes responsible for the future growth and development of the fetus, including reproductive capacity. Cell biology is concerned with the physiological properties, metabolic processes, signalling pathways, life cycle, chemical composition and interactions of cells with their environment. Cell biology involves genetics, biochemistry, molecular biology, immunology and cytochemistry. Human cells are eukaryotes - they contain organelles. The generalized structure of a eukaryotic cell is shown in Figure 2.

Figure 2. A diagram of a mammalian cell

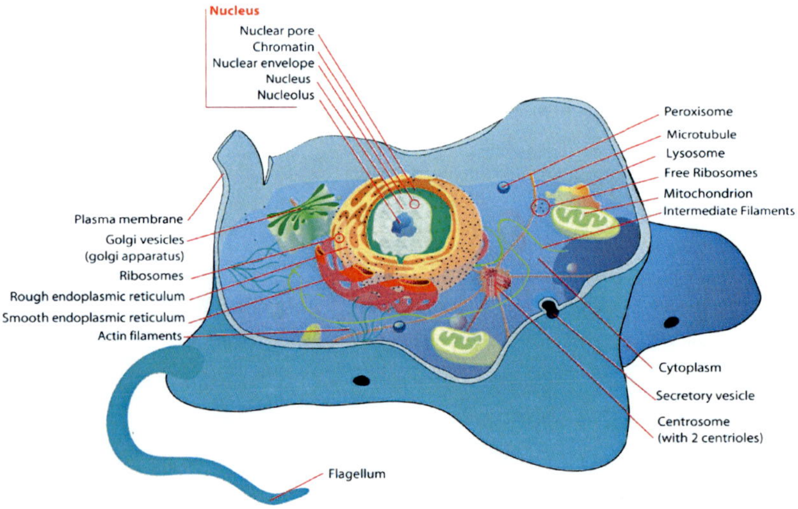

Most of the processes of eukaryotic cells are performed by a mixture of small organic molecules, inorganic ions, hormones and water. Approximately 75-85% of the cell's volume is due to water making it an indispensable solvent as a result of its polarity and structure. The shape of cells are generally round and spherical or oval.

The main constituents of the cell include proteins and lipids which are either free-flowing or membrane-bound, along with different internal compartments known as organelles. The cytoplasm is all of the material within a cell, enclosed by the cell membrane, except for the cell nucleus. The material inside the nucleus and contained within the nuclear membrane is termed the nucleoplasm. A cell's DNA, contained on the cell's chromosomes, is located within the cell's nucleus. The main components of the cytoplasm are cytosol – a gel-like substance, the organelles – the cell's internal sub-structures - and various cytoplasmic inclusions. Cell are composed of hydrophilic and hydrophobic regions. The hydrophilic regions of the cell are on both the inside and outside of the cell, while the hydrophobic regions are within the phospholipid bilayer of the cell membrane. A diagram of a mammalian cell membrane is shown in Figure 3. This shows the detailed diagram of lipid bilayer cell membrane. The cell membrane, also called the plasma membrane or plasmalemma, biological molecules, primarily proteins and lipids, which are involved in a vast array of cellular processes. It also serves as the attachment point for both the intracellular cytoskeleton and, if present, the cell wall.

Figure 3.

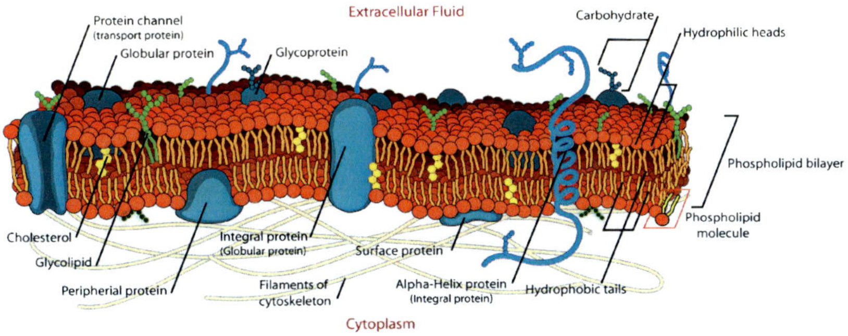

This image has been released into the public domain by its author, LadyofHats (Mariana Ruiz). Source: Own work. Image renamed from File:Cell membrane detailed diagram.svg. https://commons.wikimedia.org/wiki/File:Cell_membrane_detailed_diagram_en.svg. No changes have been made to this image.

In order for molecules to participate in reactions within the cell, they need to be able to cross this membrane layer to get into the cell. They accomplish this process of gaining access to the cell via osmotic pressure, diffusion, concentration gradients, and membrane channels. Inside the cell are extensive internal suB cellular membrane-bounded compartments called organelles.

Figure 4. Some of the cell surface proteins and internal signalling pathways of a normal human cell.

This image is in the public domain in the United States because it is a work prepared by an officer or employee of the United States Government as part of that person's official duties under the terms of Title 17, Chapter 1, Section 105 of the US Code. Source: http://dir.niehs.nih.gov/dirlst/imagemap/cell.jpg. https://commons.wikimedia.org/wiki/File:NIEHScell.jpg. No changes have been made to this image.

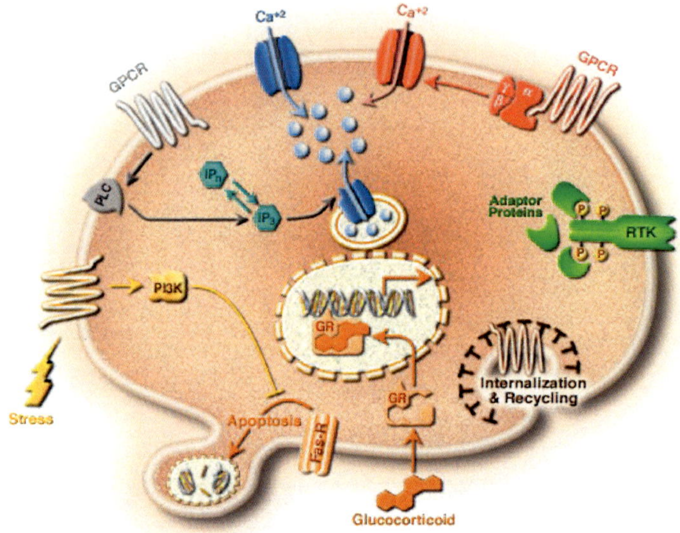

Cell growth pertains to the increase in the number of cells present in an organism as it grows and develops; in order for the organism to grow the number of cells present must increase. To enable cell growth and development the cell goes through the steps of the cell cycle: DNA replication, cell division, regeneration, specialization, and cell death. The cell cycle is divided into four distinct phases, G1, S, G2, and M. The G phases (cell growth) make up approximately 95% of the cycle. After proliferation cells then differentiate to become specialized in order to form specialized tissues, then organs and ultimately systems. The G phases along with the S phase – DNA replication, damage and repair - are considered to be the interphase portion of the cycle. While the M phase (mitosis and cytokinesis) is the cell division portion of the cycle. The cell cycle is regulated by a series of signalling factors and complexes such as cyclin-dependent kinases and p53. When the cell has completed its growth process, and if it is found to be damaged or altered, it undergoes cell death, either by apoptosis or necrosis, in order to eliminate the threat it can cause to the organism's survival. Some of the main cell surface proteins and internal signalling processes are shown in Figure 3.

Essential cell processes include

- Active transport and passive transport – the movement of molecules into and out of cells

- Adhesion - holding cells and tissues together
- Cell movement - chemotaxis, contraction and cilia
- Cell signalling - regulation of cell behaviour by signals from outside and inside the cell
- Division – the process by which cells reproduce either by mitosis (to produce clones of the parent cell) or meiosis (to produce haploid gametes either male [sperm)] or female [ova]) dependent on the gender of the organism
- DNA repair - cell death and cell senescence
- Metabolism - glycolysis, respiration, photosynthesis, and chemosynthesis
- Signal transduction - the process by which the activities in the cell are regulated
- Transcription and mRNA splicing - gene expression

Three of the most important processes – signal transduction, gene expression and apoptosis (also known as programmed cell death) - are described furtherl below. Some of the most important pathways for understanding the basis of targeted therapies, such as the pathways for angiogenesis, interkeukin (IL) 4, IL-12 and IL-23 and the TNF pathways are described in chapters dealing with the therapeutic use of molecules involved in these pathways.

Signal transduction and cell signalling pathways

Signal transduction is the process by which a chemical or physical signal is transmitted through a cell as a series of molecular events, most commonly protein phosphorylation catalyzed by protein kinases, which ultimately results in a cellular response. Proteins responsible for detecting stimuli such as ligands are termed receptors The changes elicited by ligand binding to a receptor give rise to a biochemical cascade otherwise known as a signalling path.

; https://en.wikipedia.org/wiki/Creative_Commons_license. No changes have been made to the image

When signalling pathways interact with one another they form networks, which allow cellular responses to be coordinated, often by combinatorial signalling events. At the molecular level, such responses include changes in the transcription or translation of genes, and post-translational and conformational changes in proteins, as well as changes in their location. These molecular events are the basic mechanisms controlling cell growth, proliferation, metabolism and many other processes. In multicellular organisms, signal transduction pathways have evolved to regulate cell communication in a wide variety of ways.

Each component (or node) of a signalling pathway is classified according to the role it plays with respect to the initial stimulus. Ligands are termed first messengers, while receptors are the signal transducers, which then activate primary effectors. Such effectors are often linked to second messengers, which can activate secondary effectors, and so on. Depending on the efficiency of the nodes, a signal can be amplified (a concept known as signal gain), so that one signalling molecule can generate a response involving hundreds to millions of molecules With the advent of computational biology, the analysis of signalling pathways and networks has become an essential tool to understand cellular functions and disease, including signalling rewiring mechanisms underlying responses to acquired drug resistance.

Ligands

The majority of signal transduction pathways involve the binding of signalling molecules, known as ligands, to receptors that trigger events inside the cell. The binding of a signalling molecule with a receptor causes a change in the conformation of the receptor, known as receptor activation. Most ligands are soluble molecules from the extracellular medium which bind to cell surface receptors. These include growth factors, cytokines and neurotransmitters. Components of the extracellular matrix such as fibronectin and hyaluronan can also bind to such receptors (integrins and CD44, respectively). In addition, some molecules such as steroid hormones are lipid-soluble and thus cross the plasma membrane to reach nuclear receptors.

Some receptors such as HER2/neu are capable of ligand-independent activation when overexpressed or mutated. This leads to constitutive activation of the pathway, which may or may not be overturned by compensation mechanisms. In the case of HER2, which acts as a dimerization partner of other EGFRs, constitutive activation leads to hyperproliferation and cancer – primarily some cases of breast cancer and gastric cancer (HER2/neu is also known as receptor tyrosine-protein kinase erbB-2, CD340, proto-oncogene Neu and ERBB2). A ribbon diagram of the Fab fragment of trastuzumab, a monoclonal antibody, bound to the extracellular domain of HER2 is shown in Figure 5.

Figure 5

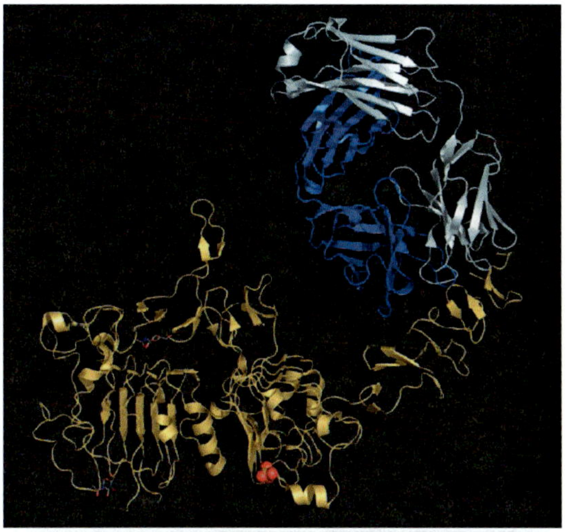

Ribbon diagram of the Fab fragment of trastuzumab, a monoclonal antibody, bound to the extracellular domain of HER2. Legend: Trastuzumab Fab fragment, heavy chain ; Trastuzumab Fab fragment, light chain ; HER2, extracellular domain

https://commons.wikimedia.org/wiki/File:Trastuzumab_Fab-HER2_complex_1N8Z.png#/media/File:Trastuzumab_Fab-HER2_complex_1N8Z.png; https://commons.wikimedia.org/wiki/User:Fvasconcellos. Created using Accelrys DS Visualizer Pro 1.6 and GIMP. More information: Cho HS, Mason K, Ramyar KX, et al. (2003). "Structure of the extracellular region of HER2 alone and in complex with the Herceptin Fab". Nature 421 (6924): 756–60. PMID 12610629. doi:10.1038/nature01392. No changes have been made to this image.

Extracellular receptors, ligand binding, messengers and adaptor proteins

Extracellular receptors are integral transmembrane proteins that span the plasma membrane (Figure 2) of the cell, with one part of the receptor on the outside of the cell and the other on the inside. Signal transduction occurs as a result of a ligand binding to the outside region of the receptor (the ligand does not pass through the membrane). Ligand-receptor binding induces a change in the conformation of the inside part of the receptor, a process sometimes called "receptor activation". This results in either the activation of an enzyme domain of the receptor or the exposure of a binding site for other intracellular signalling proteins within the cell, eventually propagating the signal through the cytoplasm (Figure 5).

In mammalian cells most intracellular proteins activated by a ligand/receptor interaction possess an enzymatic activity; examples include tyrosine kinases and phosphatases. Often such enzymes are covalently linked to the receptor. Some of them create second messengers such as cyclic AMP and IP3, the latter controlling the release of intracellular calcium stores into the cytoplasm. Other activated proteins interact with adaptor proteins (an example is shown Figure 4) that facilitate signalling protein interactions and coordination of signalling complexes necessary to respond to a particular stimulus. Enzymes and adaptor proteins are both responsive to various second messenger molecules.

Many adaptor proteins and enzymes activated as part of signal transduction possess specialized protein domains that bind to specific secondary messenger molecules. For example, calcium ions bind to the EF hand domains of calmodulin, allowing it to bind and activate calmodulin-dependent kinase.

The following major extracellular receptor/ligand binding pathways will be discussed in more detail below:

- G protein-coupled receptors
- Tyrosine, seronine/threonine- and histidine-specific protein kinases
- Integrins
- Toll-like receptors
- Ligand-gated ion binding channels

G proteins, also known as guanine nucleotide-binding proteins, are a family of proteins that act as molecular switches inside cells, and are involved in transmitting signals from a variety of stimuli outside a cell to its interior. Their activity is regulated by factors that control their ability to bind to and hydrolyze guanosine triphosphate (GTP) to guanosine diphosphate (GDP). When they are bound to GTP, they are 'on', and, when they are bound to GDP, they are 'off'.

They possess seven transmembrane domains and are linked to a heterotrimeric G protein. A ribbon diagram of a G protein is shown in Figure 7. Beta and gamma subunits of G-protein are shown by blue and red, respectively, in the phosducin-transducin beta-gamma complex. (Phosducin binds tightly to the beta gamma subunits (Gt beta gamma) of the heterotrimeric G protein transducin, preventing Gt beta gamma reassociation with Gt alpha-GDP and thereby inhibiting the G-protein cycle).

Figure 6. Ribbon diagram of a G protein

This image has been released into the public domain by its creator, Andrei Lomize, has placed it there. By Andrei Lomize - Own work, Public Domain,

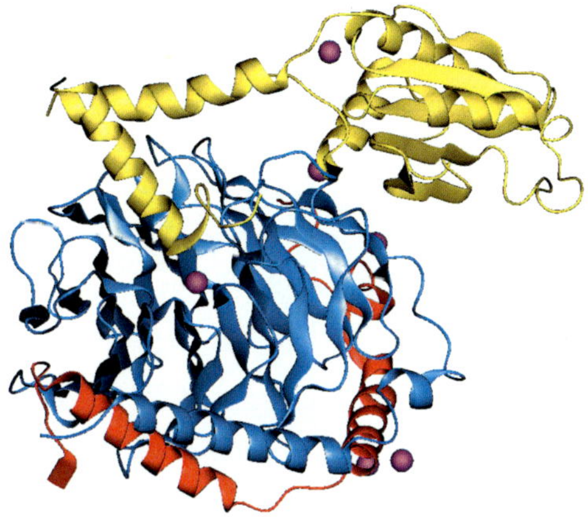

Tyrosine and seronine/threonine-specific protein kinases

Receptor tyrosine kinases (RTKs) are transmembrane proteins with an intracellular kinase domain and an extracellular domain that binds ligands (Figure 4); examples include growth factor receptors such as the insulin receptor. To perform signal transduction, RTKs need to form dimers in the plasma membrane. The dimer is stabilized by ligands binding to the receptor. The interaction between the cytoplasmic domains stimulates the autophosphorylation of tyrosine residues within the intracellular kinase domains of the RTKs, causing conformational changes. Subsequent to this, the receptors' kinase domains are activated, initiating phosphorylation signalling cascades of downstream cytoplasmic molecules that facilitate various cellular processes such as cell differentiation and metabolism. Many serine/threonine and dual-specificity protein kinases are important for signal transduction, either acting downstream of receptor tyrosine kinases, or as membrane-embedded or cell-soluble versions in their own right. The process of signal transduction involves around 560 known protein kinases and pseudokinanases, encoded by the human kinome. The kinome of an organism is the complete set of protein kinases encoded in its genome.

As is the case with GPCRs, proteins that bind GTP play a major role in signal transduction from the activated RTK into the cell. In this case, the G proteins are members of the Ras, Rho (see Figure 4 above), and Raf families, referred to collectively as small G proteins. They act as molecular switches usually tethered to membranes by isoprenyl groups linked to their carboxyl ends. Upon activation, they assign proteins to specific membrane subdomains where they participate in signalling. Activated RTKs in turn activate small G proteins that activate guanine nucleotide exchange factors such as SOS1. Once activated, these exchange factors can activate more small G proteins, thus amplifying the receptor's initial signal. The mutation of certain RTK genes, as with that of GPCRs, can result in the expression of receptors that exist in a constitutively activated state. Such mutated genes may act as oncogenes. An example is the BCR-ABL gene, which is translated to the BCR-ABL protein, a growth factor responsible for the development of chronic myeloid leukemia (CML). The first tyrosine kinase inhibitor developed that was therapeutically successful is imatinib, now routinely used as first-line treatment of CML, obviating the need in many cases of the only curative treatment for CML – allogeneic hematopoietic stem cell transplantaion, a procedure that had a treatment-related mortality of 20-30%.

Integrins

Integrins are produced by a wide variety of cells. They play a role in cell attachment to other cells and the extracellular matrix and in the transduction of signals from extracellular matrix components such as fibronectin and collagen (Figure 7).

Figure 7. An overview of integrin-mediated signal transduction, adapted from Hehlgens et al. (2007).

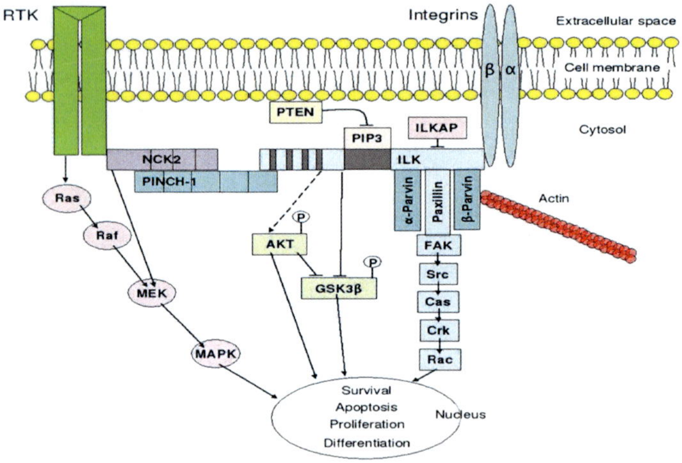

This image has been released into the public domain by its author, K.murphy at English Wikipedia. https://commons.wikimedia.org/wiki/File:Integrin_sig_trans_overview.jpeg. Original source: Hehlgans S, Haase M, Cordes N (Jan 2007). "Signalling via integrins: implications for cell survival and anticancer strategies". Biochimica et Biophysica Acta. 1775 (1): 163–80. doi:10.1016/j.bbcan.2006.09.001. PMID 17084981.

Ligand binding to the extracellular domain of integrins changes the protein's conformation, clustering it at the cell membrane to initiate signal transduction. Integrins lack kinase activity; hence, integrin-mediated signal transduction is achieved through a variety of intracellular protein kinases and adaptor molecules, the main coordinator being integrin-linked kinase. As shown in Figure 7, cooperative integrin-RTK signalling determines the timing of cellular survival, apoptosis, proliferation and differentiation.

Toll-like receptors

When activated, toll-like receptors (TLRs) take adapter molecules within the cytoplasm of cells in order to propagate a signal.

Four adaptor molecules are known to be involved in signalling. These are Myd88, TIRAP, TRIF, and TRAM. These adapter molecules activate other intracellular molecules such as IRAK1, IRAK4, TBK1, and IKKi that amplify the signal, eventually leading to the induction or suppression of genes that cause certain responses. Thousands of genes are activated by TLR signalling, implying that this method constitutes an important gateway for gene modulation.

Messenger systems

First messengers are the signalling molecules (hormones, neurotransmitters and paracrine/autocrine agents) that reach the cell from the extracellular fluid and bind to their specific receptors.

Second messengers are the substances that enter the cytoplasm and act within the cell to trigger a response. Second messengers serve as chemical relays from the plasma membrane to the cytoplasm, thus carrying out intracellular signal transduction.

Calcium

The release of calcium ions from the endoplasmic reticulum (Figure 1) into the cytosol results in its binding to signalling proteins that are then activated. It is then sequestered in the smooth endoplasmic reticulum and the mitochondria (Figure 1). Calcium is used in many processes including muscle contraction, neurotransmitter release from nerve endings, and cell migration. The three main pathways that lead to its activation are GPCR pathways, RTK pathways, and gated ion channels. It regulates proteins either directly or by binding to an enzyme.

Cellular responses

Gene activations and metabolism alterations are examples of cellular responses to extracellular stimulation that require signal transduction. Gene activation leads to further cellular effects, since the products of responding genes include instigators of activation. Transcription factors produced as a result of a signal transduction cascade can activate even more genes. Hence, an initial stimulus can trigger the expression of a large number of genes, leading to physiological events. Examples are the increased uptake of glucose from the blood stream and the migration of neutrophils to sites of infection.

Mammalian cells require stimulation for cell division and survival. In the absence of growth factor, apoptosis (programmed cell death – see below) ensues. Such requirements for extracellular stimulation are necessary for controlling cell behavior. Signal transduction pathways are perceived to be so central to biological processes that a large number of diseases are attributed to their dysregulation. Three basic types of signals determine cellular growth:

1. Stimulatory signals (growth factors)

Transcription-dependent response
Steroids are an example of this. They bind DNA, which needs to be transcribed. The produced mRNA needs to be translated, and the produced protein/peptide can undergo posttranslational modification (PMT).

Transcription-independent response
Epidermal growth factor (EGF) is an example. It binds to the epidermal growth factor receptor (EGFR), which causes dimerization and autophosphorylation of the EGFR, which in turn activates the intracellular signalling pathway.

2. Inhibitory signals (cell-cell contact)

3. Permissive signals (cell-matrix interactions)

The combination of these signals are integrated in an altered cytoplasmic machinery which leads to altered cell behaviour.

Major cell signalling pathways
The following are some of the major cell signalling pathways, demonstrating how ligands binding to their receptors can affect second messengers and eventually result in altered cellular responses.

- MAPK/ERK pathway: a pathway that couples intracellular responses to the binding of growth factors to cell surface receptors. This pathway is very complex and includes many protein components. In many cell types, activation of this pathway promotes cell division, and many forms of cancer are associated with aberrations in it.
- cAMP-dependent pathway: cAMP works by activating protein kinase A (PKA, cAMP-dependent protein kinase (Figure 11). Further effects depend mainly on cAMP-dependent protein kinase, which vary based on the type of cell involved.
- IP3/DAG pathway: PLC cleaves the phospholipid phosphatidylinositol 4,5-bisphosphate (PIP2), yielding diacyl glycerol (DAG) and inositol 1,4,5-triphosphate (IP3). DAG remains bound to the

membrane, and IP3 is released as a soluble structure into the cytosol. IP3 then diffuses through the cytosol to bind to IP3 receptors, particular calcium channels in the endoplasmic reticulum (ER). These channels are specific to calcium and allow the passage of only calcium to move through. This causes the cytosolic concentration of calcium to increase, in turn precipitating a cascade of intracellular changes and activity. In addition, calcium and DAG together work to activate PKC, which then phosphorylates other molecules, leading to altered cellular activity.

DNA, RNA and genes

DNA is a molecule composed of two chains that coil around each other to form a double helix carrying the genetic instructions used in the growth, development, functioning, and reproduction of all known organisms and many viruses. DNA and ribonucleic acid (RNA) are nucleic acids. Nucleic acids, together with proteins, lipids and complex carbohydrates (polysaccharides), are one of the four major types of macromolecules that are essential for all known forms of life.

The two DNA strands are also known as polynucleotides as they are composed of simpler monomeric units called nucleotides. Each nucleotide is composed of one of four nitrogen-containing nucleobases (cytosine [C], guanine [G], adenine [A] or thymine [T]), a sugar called deoxyribose, and a phosphate group.

Figure 8 is a graphic of DNA replication. The nitrogenous bases of the two separate polynucleotide strands are bound together, according to base pairing rules (A with T and C with G), with hydrogen bonds to make double-stranded DNA in a helical form.

Figure 8. A graphic of DNA replication.

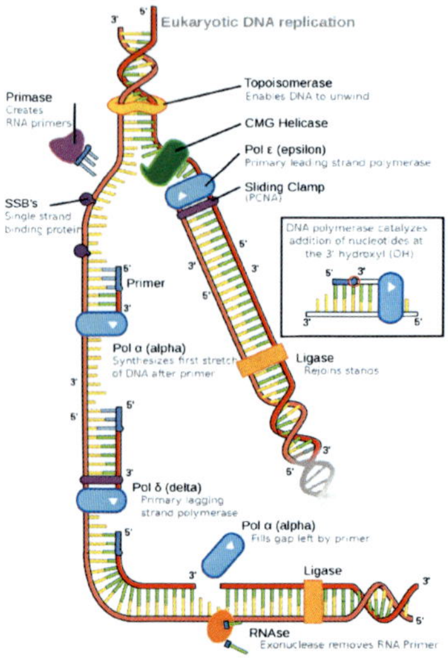

Genes

A gene is a sequence of nucleotides in DNA or RNA that codes for a molecule that has a function. Genes are contained on the chromosomes in the cell nucleus. During gene expression, the DNA is first copied into RNA. The RNA can be directly functional or be the intermediate template for a protein that performs a function. A chromosome consists of a long strand of DNA containing many genes. A human chromosome can have up to 500 million base pairs of DNA with thousands of genes. Gene expression is the process by which information from a gene is used in the synthesis of a functional gene product. These products are often proteins, When the end-product is a protein, genes are first transcribed into RNA, and this transcript is then translated into protein. Several steps in the gene expression process may be modulated, including transcription, RNA splicing, translation and post-translational modification of the protein. Gene regulation gives the cell control over structure and function, and is the basis for cellular differentiation, morphogenesis and the versatility and adaptability of any organism.

Genes are expressed by being transcribed into RNA, and this transcript may then be translated into protein.

Figure 9. Diagram showing how translation of messenger RNA and protein synthesis takes place in ribosomes.

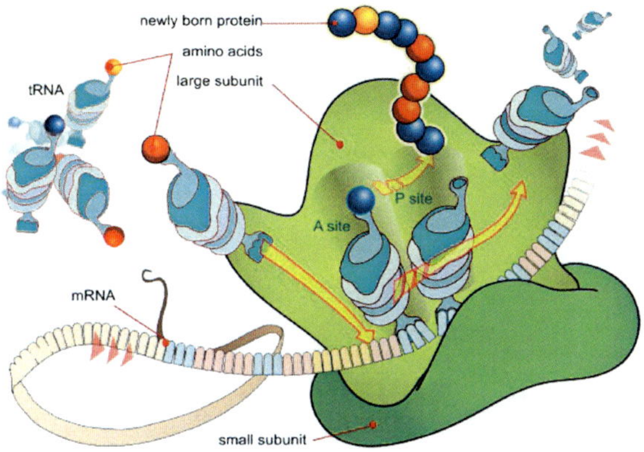

Figure 11. This work has been released into the public domain by its author, LadyofHats. By LadyofHats - Own work based on:[1], [2], [3], [4], [5], [6], [7], and [8]., Public Domain, https://commons.wikimedia.org/w/index.php?curid=4889777; https://en.wikipedia.org/wiki/Translation_(biology)#/media/File:Ribosome_mRNA_translation_en.svg. No changes have been made to this image.

Protein folding

A polypeptide (protein) folds into its characteristic and functional three-dimensional structure from a random coil. Each protein exists as an unfolded polypeptide or random coil when translated from a sequence of messenger (m) RNA into a linear chain of amino acids (Figure 10, left hand image). Amino acids interact with each other to produce a well-defined three-dimensional structure.

Figure 10 shows a protein before (left) and after (right) folding

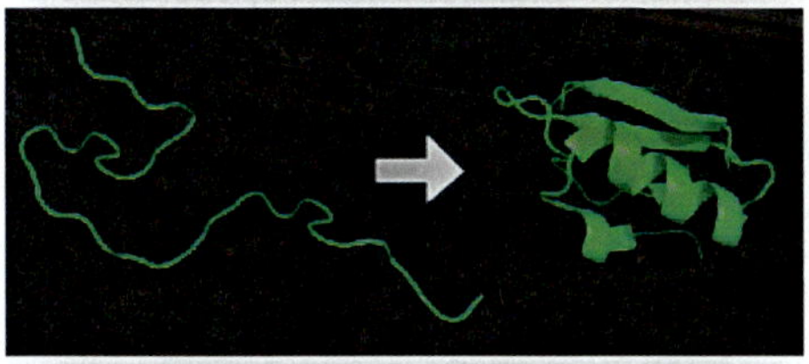

This image, reproduced here from Wikimedia Commons, is in the public domain because its creator has placed it there. By No machine-readable author provided. Dr Kjaergaard assumed (based on copyright claims). - No machine-readable source

4. The biology of malignant human cells.

Defects in genes (DNA), epigenetic factors and mismatch repair systems can all cause human cells to become malignant.

Genes

With the exception of congenital disorders, malignant human cells have an abnormality of their genetic systems, and differ in this regard to abnormal, but non-malignant, as well as to normal human cells. Carcinogenesis is the formation of a cancer, whereby normal cells are transformed into cancer cells. The process is characterized by changes at the cellular, genetic, and epigenetic levels and abnormal cell division. Cell division is a physiological process that occurs in almost all tissues and under a variety of circumstances. Normally the balance between proliferation and programmed cell death, in the form of apoptosis, is maintained to ensure the integrity of tissues and organs. According to the prevailing accepted theory of carcinogenesis, the somatic mutation theory, mutations in DNA and epimutations that lead to cancer disrupt these orderly processes by disrupting the programming regulating the processes, upsetting the normal balance between proliferation and cell death. This results in uncontrolled cell division and the evolution of those cells by natural selection in the body. Only certain mutations lead to cancer whereas the majority of mutations do not.

A series of several mutations to certain classes of genes is usually required before a normal cell will transform into a malignant cell.

In order for a normal cell to transform into a malignant cell, the genes that regulate cell growth and differentiation must be altered.

The affected genes are divided into two broad categories. Oncogenes are genes that promote cell growth and reproduction. Tumor suppressor genes are genes that inhibit cell division and survival. Malignant transformation can occur through the formation of novel oncogenes, the inappropriate over-expression of normal oncogenes, or by the under-expression or disabling of tumor suppressor genes. Typically, changes in multiple genes are required to transform a normal cell into a cancer cell (Figure 11)

Figure 11 illustrates that cancers are caused by a series of mutations. Each mutation alters the behavior of the cell to some extent.

Institute, Public Domain, https://commons.wikimedia.org/w/index.php?curid=1972023. No changes have been made to this image.

Figure 11.

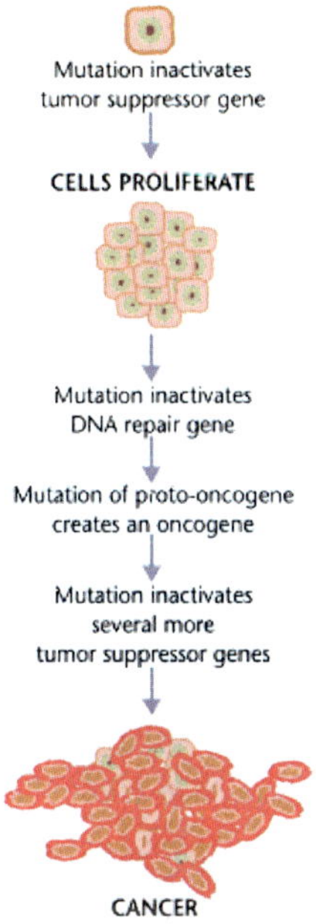

The abnormal biological properties of human malignant cells can be summarized as follows:

- Acquisition of self-sufficiency in growth signals, leading to unchecked growth.
- Loss of sensitivity to anti-growth signals, also leading to unchecked growth.
- Loss of capacity for apoptosis, allowing growth despite genetic errors and external anti-growth signals.
- Loss of capacity for senescence, leading to limitless replicative potential (immortality).
- Acquisition of sustained angiogenesis, allowing the tumor to grow beyond the limitations of passive nutrient diffusion.
- Acquisition of ability to invade neighbouring tissues, the defining property of invasive carcinoma.

- Acquisition of ability to seed metastases at distant sites, a late-appearing property of some malignant tumors (carcinomas or others).

Involved in these steps is

- Loss of capacity to repair genetic errors, leading to an increased mutation rate (genomic instability), thus accelerating all the above changes.

Often, the multiple genetic changes that result in cancer may take many years to accumulate. During this time, the biological behavior of the pre-malignant cells slowly changes from the properties of normal cells to those with cancer-like properties (Figure 12).

Figure 12 shows that tissue can be organized in a continuous spectrum from normal to malignant.

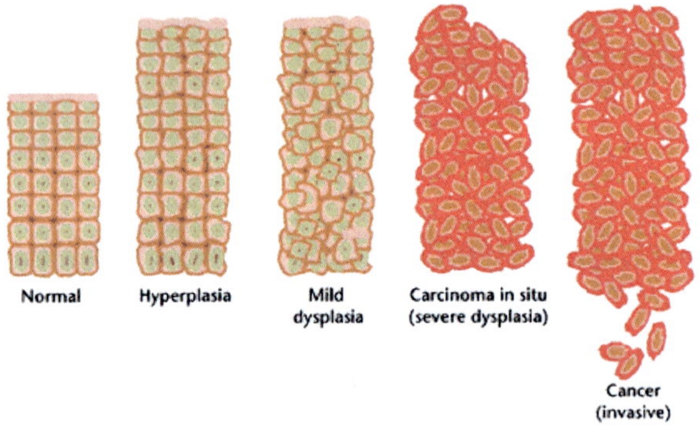

Epigenetic factors also plays a major role in the development of human cancers.

Epigenetic modifications to the DNA of cancer cells do not involve a change in the nucleotide sequence, but instead involve a change in the way the genetic code is expressed. Epigenetic alterations may be just as important, or even more important, than genetic mutations in a cell's transformation to malignancy. In malignant cells loss of expression of genes occurs about 10 times more frequently by transcription silencing (caused by epigenetic promoter hypermethylation of CpG islands) than by mutations. In different types of cancer, a variety of epigenetic mechanisms can be perturbed, such as silencing of tumor suppressor genes and activation of oncogenes by altered CpG island methylation patterns, histone modifications, and dysregulation of DNA-binding proteins.

DNA mismatch repair systems

If DNA repair is deficient, DNA damage tends to accumulate. Such excess DNA damage can increase mutational errors during DNA replication. Excess DNA damage can also increase epigenetic alterations due to errors during DNA repair. Such mutations and epigenetic alterations can give rise to malignancy. Germ line mutations in DNA repair genes cause only 2–5% of colon cancer cases. However, altered expression of microRNAs, causing DNA repair deficiencies, are frequently associated with cancers and may be an important causal factor for such cancers.

In non-hereditary cancers, a deficiency in DNA repair is occasionally found to be due to a mutation in a DNA repair gene, but reduced or absent expression of DNA repair genes is much more frequently due to epigenetic alterations that reduce or silence gene expression.

Cancer therapy procedures such as chemotherapy and radiotherapy work by overwhelming the capacity of the malignant cells to repair DNA damage, resulting in their death. Cells that are most rapidly dividing – most typically cancer cells – are preferentially affected. An important side-effect is that other non-cancerous but rapidly dividing cells such as progenitor cells in the gut, skin, and hematopoietic system are also affected. Modern cancer treatments attempt to localize the DNA damage to cells and tissues only associated with cancer, either by physical means (concentrating the therapeutic agent in the region of the tumor) or by biochemical means (exploiting a feature unique to cancer cells in the body).

5. Overview of B cell acute lymphoblastic leukemia

B cell acute lymphoblastic leukemia (ALL) is a cancer of precursor B lymphocytes in the bone marrow characterized by the development of large numbers of lymphoblasts. Symptoms may include feeling tired, pale skin color, fever, easy bleeding or bruising, enlarged lymph nodes, or bone pain. ALL progresses rapidly, metastasizes widely including into the central nervous system and is typically fatal within weeks or months if left untreated. In most cases, the cause is unknown. .

Over the past several decades, there have been strides to increase the efficacy of treatment regimens, resulting in increased survival rates. The aim of treatment is to induce a lasting remission, defined as the absence of detectable leukemia cells in the body (usually less than 5% blast cells in the bone marrow). ALL is typically treated initially with chemotherapy aimed at inducing remission. This is then followed by further chemotherapy typically over a number of years. Treatment usually also includes intrathecal chemotherapy since systemic chemotherapy has limited penetration into the central nervous system and the central nervous system is a common site for relapse of acute lymphoblastic leukemia. Treatment can also include radiation therapy if spread to the brain has occurred. Allogeneic hematopoietic stem cell transplantation may be used if the disease recurs following standard treatment. Additional treatments such as chimeric antigen receptor (CAR) T cell immunotherapy are now being used and 2 such medications have been approved by the USA FDA for relapsed or refractory B cell ALL.

ALL affected about 876,000 people globally in 2015 and resulted in about 111,000 deaths. It occurs most commonly in children, particularly those between the ages of two and five. In the United States it is the most common cause of cancer and death from cancer among children. ALL is notable for being the first disseminated cancer to be cured. Survival for children increased from under 10% in the 1960s to 90% in 2015. Survival rates remain lower for babies (50%) and adults (35%).

6. The Philadelphia chromosome

The Philadelphia chromosome or Philadelphia translocation (Ph) is a specific genetic abnormality in chromosome 22 of leukemia cancer cells.This chromosome is defective and unusually short because of reciprocal translocation, t(9;22)(q34;q11), of genetic material between chromosome 9 and chromosome 22, and contains a fusion gene called BCR-ABL1. This gene is the ABL1 gene of chromosome 9 juxtaposed onto the breakpoint cluster region BCR gene of chromosome 22, coding for a hybrid protein: a tyrosine kinase signaling protein that is "always on", causing the cell to divide uncontrollably by interrupting the stability of the genome and impairing various signaling pathways governing the cell cycle.

This translocation occurs most commonly in chronic myeloid leukemia but also occurs in a minority of 25–30% of adult cases and 2–10% of pediatric cases) in acute lymphoblastic leukemia (ALL) and is associated with a poor prognosis.

The chromosomal defect in the Philadelphia chromosome is a reciprocal translocation, in which parts of two chromosomes, 9 and 22, swap places. The result is that a fusion gene is created by juxtaposing the ABL1 gene on chromosome 9 (region q34) to a part of the BCR (breakpoint cluster region) gene on chromosome 22 (region q11). This is a reciprocal translocation, creating an elongated chromosome 9 (termed a derivative chromosome, or der 9), and a truncated chromosome 22 (the Philadelphia chromosome, 22q-). In agreement with the International System for Human Cytogenetic Nomenclature (ISCN), this chromosomal translocation is designated as t(9;22)(q34;q11). The symbol ABL1 is derived from Abelson, the name of a leukemia virus which carries a similar protein. The symbol BCR is derived from breakpoint cluster region, a gene which encodes a protein that acts as a guanine nucleotide exchange factor for Rho GTPase proteins

Translocation results in an oncogenic BCR-ABL1 gene fusion that can be found on the shorter derivative chromosome 22. This gene encodes for a BCR-ABL1 fusion protein. Depending on the precise location of fusion, the molecular weight of this protein can range from 185 to 210 kDa. Consequently, the hybrid BCR-ABL1 fusion protein is referred to as p210 or p185.

Three clinically important variants encoded by the fusion gene are the p190, p210, and p230 isoforms. p190 is generally associated with B-cell acute lymphoblastic leukemia (ALL), while p210 is generally associated with chronic myeloid leukemia but can also be associated with ALL and AML.

The ABL1 gene expresses a membrane-associated protein, a tyrosine kinase, and the BCR-ABL1 transcript is also translated into a tyrosine kinase containing domains from both the BCR and ABL1 genes. The activity of tyrosine kinases is typically regulated in an auto-inhibitory fashion, but the BCR-ABL1 fusion gene codes for a protein that is "always on" or constitutively activated, leading to impaired DNA binding and unregulated cell division (i.e. cancer). This is due to the replacement of the myristoylated cap region, which when present induces a conformational change rendering the kinase domain inactive, with a truncated portion of the BCR protein.

The fused BCR-ABL1 protein interacts with the interleukin-3 receptor beta(c) subunit and is moderated by an activation loop within its SH1 domain, which is turned "on" when bound to ATP and triggers downstream pathways. The ABL1 tyrosine kinase activity of BCR-ABL1 is elevated relative to wild-type ABL1. Since ABL activates a number of cell cycle-controlling proteins and enzymes, the result of the BCR-ABL1 fusion is to speed up cell division. Moreover, it inhibits DNA repair, causing genomic instability.

7. Overview of conventional treatment of ALL

Successful treatment of acute lymphoblastic leukemia (ALL) consists of the control of bone marrow and systemic disease and the treatment (or prevention) of sanctuary-site disease, particularly the central nervous system (CNS). The cornerstone of this strategy includes systemically administered combination chemotherapy with CNS preventive therapy. CNS prophylaxis is achieved with chemotherapy (intrathecal and/or high-dose systemic therapy) and, in some cases, cranial radiation therapy.

Treatment is divided into the following three phases:

Remission induction.

Central Nervous System (CNS) prophylaxis.

Postremission (also called remission continuation or maintenance).

The average length of treatment for ALL varies between 1.5 and 3 years in the effort to eradicate the leukemic cell population.

Standard Treatment Options for Adult Acute Lymphoblastic Leukemia (ALL)

Standard treatment options for untreated adult acute lymphoblastic leukemia (ALL) include the following:

Remission induction therapy, including the following:

Combination chemotherapy.

Imatinib mesylate (for patients with Philadelphia chromosome [Ph1]-positive ALL).

Imatinib mesylate combined with combination chemotherapy (for patients with Ph1-positive ALL)

Supportive care.

Central nervous system (CNS) prophylaxis therapy, which can include the following:

cranial radiation therapy plus intrathecal (IT) methotrexate.

high-dose systemic methotrexate and IT methotrexate without cranial radiation therapy.

Remission induction therapy

Sixty percent to 80% of adults with ALL usually achieve a complete remission status following appropriate induction therapy. Appropriate initial treatment, usually consisting of a regimen that includes the combination of vincristine, prednisone, and an anthracycline, with or without asparaginase, results in a complete response rate of up to 80%. In patients with Ph1-positive ALL, the remission rate is generally greater than 90% when standard induction regimens are combined with BCR-ABL tyrosine kinase inhibitors. In the largest study published to date of Ph1-positive ALL patients, 1,913 adult patients with ALL had a 5-year overall survival (OS) rate of 39%.

Patients who experience a relapse after remission usually die within 1 year, even if a second complete remission is achieved. If there are appropriate available donors and if the patient is younger than 55 years, hematopoietic stem cell transplantation (HSCT) may be a consideration in the management of this disease. Transplant centers performing five or fewer transplants annually usually have poorer results than larger centers. If allogeneic transplant is considered, a recommendation is that transfusions with blood products from a potential donor be avoided, if possible.

Combination chemotherapy

Most current induction regimens for patients with adult ALL include combination chemotherapy with prednisone, vincristine, and an anthracycline. Some regimens, including those used in a Cancer and Leukemia Group B (CALGB) study (CLB-8811), also add other drugs, such as asparaginase or cyclophosphamide. Current multiagent induction regimens result in complete response rates that range from 60% to 90%.

Imatinib mesylate

Imatinib mesylate is often incorporated into the therapeutic plan for patients with Ph1-positive ALL. Imatinib mesylate, an orally available inhibitor of the BCR-ABL tyrosine kinase, has been shown to have clinical activity as a single agent in Ph1-positive ALL. More commonly, particularly in younger patients, imatinib is incorporated into combination chemotherapy regimens. There are several published single-arm studies in which the complete response rate and survival are compared with historical controls.

Several studies have suggested that the addition of imatinib to conventional combination chemotherapy induction regimens results in complete response rates, event-free survival rates, and OS rates that are higher than those in historical controls. At the present time, no conclusions can be drawn regarding the optimal imatinib dose or schedule.

In a study of imatinib combined with chemotherapy from the Northern Italy Leukemia Group, patients with newly diagnosed, untreated Ph1-positive ALL were treated with an induction regimen containing idarubicin, vincristine, prednisone, and L-asparaginase. After accrual of an initial cohort, the study was modified to include the use of imatinib (600 mg qd from days 15 to 21). In consolidation, patients received imatinib (600 mg qd for 7 days) beginning 3 days before the start of each course of chemotherapy.

For all patients who achieved remission, the intent was to proceed to an allogeneic HSC transplant. when and if, an HLA-matched donor could be identified. Patients lacking a donor received an autologous transplant. After completion of chemotherapy and transplant, all patients were to receive maintenance imatinib for as long as tolerated. After 20 patients had accrued to the imatinib arm, L-asparaginase was omitted from the induction regimen from both arms because of toxicity.

Outcomes for the first cohort of 35 patients (imatinib-free) were compared with those of the subsequent cohort of 59 (imatinib-treated) patients. For patients treated with imatinib, OS probability was 38% at 5 years (median, 3.1 year) versus 23% in the imatinib-free group (median, 1.1 year; P = .009).

The drawbacks of this nonrandomized study are the small sample size (94 total patients) and the change in the treatment regimen (omission of L-asparaginase) midway through the study. However, the results suggest that inclusion of imatinib into a relatively standard chemotherapy regimen for newly diagnosed adult patients with Ph1-positive ALL may provide a significant survival advantage.

In another study, ten patients with Ph1-positive ALL and ten patients with chronic myelogenous leukemia in lymphoid blast crisis were treated with doses of imatinib ranging from 300 mg to 1,000 mg per day. Of these 20 patients, four had complete hematologic remission and ten had marrow responses. Responses were short lived, with most of these patients experiencing disease relapse at a median of 58 days after the start of therapy.

In another study, 48 patients with Ph1-positive ALL were treated with 400 mg to 800 mg of imatinib per day. The overall response rate was 60%, with 9 out of 48 patients (19%) achieving a complete remission. The responses again were short, with a median duration of 2.2 months.

In each of these studies, common toxicities were nausea and liver enzyme abnormalities, which necessitated interruption and/or dose reduction of imatinib. Subsequent allogeneic transplant does not appear to be adversely affected by the addition of imatinib to the treatment regimen.

Imatinib is generally incorporated into the treatment of patients with Ph1-positive ALL because of the responses observed in monotherapy trials. If a suitable donor is available, allogeneic bone marrow transplantation should be considered because remissions are generally short with conventional ALL chemotherapy clinical trials.

Supportive care

Randomized clinical trials have shown similar outcomes for patients who received prophylactic platelet transfusions at a level of 10,000/mm^3 rather than at a level of 20,000/mm^3.

Empiric broad-spectrum antimicrobial therapy is an absolute necessity for febrile patients who are profoundly neutropenic. Careful instruction in personal hygiene and dental care and in recognizing early signs of infection are appropriate for all patients. Elaborate isolation facilities, including filtered air, sterile food, and gut flora sterilization, are not routinely indicated but may benefit transplant patients.

As suggested in a CALGB study (CLB-9111), the use of myeloid growth factors during remission-induction therapy appears to decrease the time to hematopoietic reconstitution.

CNS prophylaxis therapy

The early institution of CNS prophylaxis is critical to achieve control of sanctuary disease.

Special Considerations for B-Cell ALL

Two additional subtypes of adult ALL require special consideration. B-cell ALL, which expresses surface immunoglobulin and cytogenetic abnormalities such as t(8;14), t(2;8), and t(8;22), is not usually cured with typical ALL regimens. Aggressive, brief-duration, high-intensity regimens, including those previously used in CLB-9251 (NCT00002494), that are similar to those used in aggressive non-Hodgkin lymphoma have shown high response rates and cure rates (75% complete response; 40% failure-free survival).

9. TARGETED IMMUNE THERAPIES FOR ACUTE LYMPHOBLASTIC LEUKEMIA

This book deals only with four immunotherapeutic targeted agents that have been FDA-approved for therapeutic use in precursor B ALL. They are

Blinatumomab (Blincyto) - a bispecific monoclonal antibody directed at CD19 and CD3

Inotuzumab ozogamicin (Besponsa) - a monoclonal antibody/drug conjugate directed at CD22

Tisagenlecleucel (Kymriah) – a cell-mediated gene therapy directed at CD19

Brexucabtagene autoleucel (Tecartus) - a cell-mediated gene therapy directed at CD19

CD3 (cluster of differentiation 3) is a protein complex and T cell co-receptor that is involved in activating both the cytotoxic T cell (CD8+ naive T cells) and T helper cells (CD4+ naive T cells). It is composed of four distinct chains. In mammals, the complex contains a CD3γ chain, a CD3δ chain, and two CD3ε chains. These chains associate with the T-cell receptor (TCR) and the CD3-zeta (ζ-chain) to generate an activation signal in T lymphocytes. The TCR, CD3-zeta, and the other CD3 molecules together constitute the TCR complex.

CD19 is expressed in all human B lineage cells. Contrary to some early doubts, human plasma cells do express CD19 as confirmed by others CD19 plays two major roles in human B cells: on the one hand, it acts as an adaptor protein to recruit cytoplasmic signalling proteins to the membrane; on the other, it works within the CD19/CD21 complex to decrease the threshold for B cell receptor signalling pathways.

CD22 is found on the surface of mature human B cells and to a lesser extent on some immature B cells. Generally speaking, CD22 is a regulatory molecule that prevents the overactivation of the immune system and the development of autoimmune diseases. CD22 is a sugar binding transmembrane protein, which specifically binds sialic acid with an immunoglobulin (Ig) domain located at its N-terminus. The presence of Ig domains makes CD22 a member of the immunoglobulin superfamily. CD22 functions as an inhibitory receptor for B cell receptor (BCR) signalling.

10. BLINCYTO® (blinatumomab) for injection, for intravenous use

INDICATIONS AND USAGE

1.1. MRD-positive B-cell Precursor ALL

BLINCYTO is indicated for the treatment of

B-cell precursor acute lymphoblastic leukemia (ALL) in first or second complete remission with minimal residual disease (MRD) greater than or equal to 0.1% in adults and children.

This indication is approved under accelerated approval based on MRD response rate and hematological relapse-free survival. Continued approval for this indication may be contingent upon verification and description of clinical benefit in the confirmatory trials.

1.2. Relapsed or Refractory B-cell Precursor ALL

BLINCYTO is indicated for the treatment of relapsed or refractory B-cell precursor acute lymphoblastic leukemia (ALL) in adults and children.

2. DOSAGE AND ADMINISTRATION

2.1. Treatment of MRD-Positive B-cell Precursor ALL

A treatment course consists of 1 cycle of BLINCYTO for induction followed by up to 3 additional cycles for consolidation.

A single cycle of treatment of BLINCYTO induction or consolidation consists of 28 days of continuous intravenous infusion followed by a 14-day treatment-free interval (total 42 days).

See Table 1 for the recommended dose by patient weight and schedule. Patients greater than or equal to 45 kg receive a fixed-dose. For patients less than 45 kg, the dose is calculated using the patient's body surface area (BSA).

Table 1. Recommended BLINCYTO Dosage and Schedule for the Treatment of MRD-positive B-cell Precursor ALL

Cycle	Patient Weight Greater Than or Equal to 45 kg (Fixed-dose)	Patient Weight Less Than 45 kg (BSA-based dose)

Induction Cycle 1 Days 1-28 Days 29-42	 28 mcg/day 14-day treatment-free interval	 15 mcg/m²/day (not to exceed 28 mcg/day) 14-day treatment-free interval
Consolidation Cycles 2-4 Days 1-28 Days 29-42	 28 mcg/day 14-day treatment-free interval	 15 mcg/m²/day (not to exceed 28 mcg/day) 14-day treatment-free interval

Hospitalization is recommended for the first 3 days of the first cycle and the first 2 days of the second cycle. For all subsequent cycle starts and re-initiations (e.g., if treatment is interrupted for 4 or more hours), supervision by a healthcare professional or hospitalization is recommended.

Premedicate with prednisone or equivalent for MRD-positive B-cell Precursor ALL

For adult patients, premedicate with prednisone 100 mg intravenously or equivalent (e.g., dexamethasone 16 mg) 1 hour prior to the first dose of BLINCYTO in each cycle.

For pediatric patients, premedicate with 5 mg/m^2 of dexamethasone, to a maximum dose of 20 mg prior to the first dose of BLINCYTO in the first cycle and when restarting an infusion after an interruption of 4 or more hours in the first cycle.

For administration of BLINCYTO:

See Section 2.5 for infusion over 24 hours or 48 hours.

See Section 2.6 for infusion over 7 days using Bacteriostatic 0.9% Sodium Chloride Injection, USP (containing 0.9% benzyl alcohol). This option is available for patients weighing greater than or equal to 22 kg. It is not recommended for use in patients weighing less than 22 kg.

2.2. Treatment of Relapsed or Refractory B-cell Precursor ALL

A treatment course consists of up to 2 cycles of BLINCYTO for induction followed by 3 additional cycles for consolidation and up to 4 additional cycles of continued therapy.

A single cycle of treatment of BLINCYTO induction or consolidation consists of 28 days of continuous intravenous infusion followed by a 14-day treatment-free interval (total 42 days).

A single cycle of treatment of BLINCYTO continued therapy consists of 28 days of continuous intravenous infusion followed by a 56-day treatment-free interval (total 84 days).

See Table 2 for the recommended dose by patient weight and schedule. Patients greater than or equal to 45 kg receive a fixed-dose and for patients less than 45 kg, the dose is calculated using the patient's body surface area (BSA).

Table 2. Recommended BLINCYTO Dosage and Schedule for the Treatment of Relapsed or Refractory B-cell Precursor ALL

Cycle	**Patient Weight Greater Than or Equal to 45 kg** **(Fixed-dose)**	**Patient Weight Less Than 45 kg** **(BSA-based dose)**
Induction Cycle 1		
Days 1-7	9 mcg/day	5 mcg/m^2/day (not to exceed 9 mcg/day)
Days 8-28	28 mcg/day	15 mcg/m^2/day (not to exceed 28 mcg/day)
Days 29-42	14-day treatment-free interval	14-day treatment-free interval

Induction Cycle 2 Days 1-28 Days 29-42	 28 mcg/day 14-day treatment-free interval	 15 mcg/m^2/day (not to exceed 28 mcg/day) 14-day treatment-free interval
Consolidation Cycles 3-5 Days 1-28 Days 29-42	 28 mcg/day 14-day treatment-free interval	 15 mcg/m^2/day (not to exceed 28 mcg/day) 14-day treatment-free interval
Continued Therapy Cycles 6-9 Days 1-28 Days 29-84	28 mcg/day 56-day treatment-free interval	15 mcg/m^2/day (not to exceed 28 mcg/day) 56-day treatment-free interval

Hospitalization is recommended for the first 9 days of the first cycle and the first 2 days of the second cycle. For all subsequent cycle starts and re-initiation (e.g., if treatment is interrupted for 4 or more hours), supervision by a healthcare professional or hospitalization is recommended.

Premedicate with dexamethasone.

For adult patients, premedicate with 20 mg dexamethasone 1 hour prior to the first dose of BLINCYTO of each cycle, prior to a step dose (such as Cycle 1 Day 8), and when restarting an infusion after an interruption of 4 or more hours.

For pediatric patients, premedicate with 5 mg/m^2 of dexamethasone, to a maximum dose of 20 mg prior to the first dose of BLINCYTO in the first cycle, prior to a step dose (such as Cycle 1 Day 8), and when restarting an infusion after an interruption of 4 or more hours in the first cycle.

For administration of BLINCYTO:

See Section 2.5 for infusion over 24 hours or 48 hours.

See Section 2.6 for infusion over 7 days using Bacteriostatic 0.9% Sodium Chloride Injection, USP (containing 0.9% benzyl alcohol). This option is available for patients weighing greater than or equal to 22 kg. It is not recommended for use in patients weighing less than 22 kg.

2.3. Dosage Adjustments

If the interruption after an adverse event is no longer than 7 days, continue the same cycle to a total of

28 days of infusion inclusive of days before and after the interruption in that cycle. If an interruption due to an adverse event is longer than 7 days, start a new cycle.

Hospitalization is recommended for the first 9 days of the first cycle and the first 2 days of the second cycle. For all subsequent cycle starts and re-initiation (e.g., if treatment is interrupted for 4 or more hours), supervision by a healthcare professional or hospitalization is recommended.

Premedicate with dexamethasone.

For adult patients, premedicate with 20 mg dexamethasone 1 hour prior to the first dose of BLINCYTO of each cycle, prior to a step dose (such as Cycle 1 Day 8), and when restarting an infusion after an interruption of 4 or more hours.

For pediatric patients, premedicate with 5 mg/m^2 of dexamethasone, to a maximum dose of 20 mg prior to the first dose of BLINCYTO in the first cycle, prior to a step dose (such as Cycle 1 Day 8), and when restarting an infusion after an interruption of 4 or more hours in the first cycle.

For administration of BLINCYTO:

See Section 2.5 for infusion over 24 hours or 48 hours.

See Section 2.6 for infusion over 7 days using Bacteriostatic 0.9% Sodium Chloride Injection, USP (containing 0.9% benzyl alcohol). This option is available for patients weighing greater than or equal to 22 kg. It is not recommended for use in patients weighing less than 22 kg.

2.4. Dosage Adjustments

If the interruption after an adverse event is no longer than 7 days, continue the same cycle to a total of 28 days of infusion inclusive of days before and after the interruption in that cycle. If an interruption due to an adverse event is longer than 7 days, start a new cycle.

Table 3. Dose Modifications for Toxicity

Toxicity	Grade*	Patients Greater Than or Equal to 45 kg	Patients Less Than 45 kg
Cytokine Release Syndrome (CRS)	Grade 3	Withhold BLINCYTO until resolved, then restart BLINCYTO BLINCYTO at 9 mcg/day. Escalate to 28 mcg/day after 7 days if the the toxicity does not recur.	Withhold BLINCYTO until resolved, then restart at 5 mcg/m^2/day. Escalate to 15 mcg/m^2/day after 7 days if toxicity does not recur.
	Grade 4	Discontinue BLINCYTO permanently.	
Neurological	Seizure	Discontinue BLINCYTO permanently if more than one seizure occurs.	

Toxicity		
	Grade 3:	
	Withhold BLINCYTO until no more than Grade 1 (mild) and for at for at least 3 days, then restart	Withhold BLINCYTO until no more than Grade 1 (mild) and for at least
	BLINCYTO at 9 mcg/day	BLINCYTO at 5 $mcg/m^2/day$
	Escalate to 28 mcg/day after 7 days if the toxicity does not recur. If the toxicity occurred at 9mcg/day, or if the toxicity takes	Escalate to 15 $mcg/m^2/day$ after 7 days if the toxicity does not recur. If the toxicity occurred at 5 $mcg/m^2/day$, or if the toxicity
	more than 7 days to resolve, discontinue BLINCYTO permanently.	takes more than 7 days to resolve, discontinue BLINCYTO permanently.

Table 3. Dose Modifications for Toxicity (cont)

Toxicity	Grade*	Patients Greater Than or Equal to 45 kg	Patients Less Than 45 kg
Grade 4	Discontinue BLINCYTO permanently.		

Other Clinically Relevant Adverse Reactions	Grade 3: Withhold BLINCYTO until no more than Grade 1 (mild), then restart BLINCYTO at 9 mcg/day. Escalate to 28 mcg/day after 7 days if the toxicity does not recur. If the toxicity takes more than 14 days to resolve, discontinue BLINCYTO permanently.	Withhold BLINCYTO until no more than Grade 1 (mild), then restart BLINCYTO at 5 mcg/m^2/day. Escalate to 15 mcg/m^2/day after 7 days if the toxicity does not recur. If the toxicity takes more than 14 days to resolve, discontinue BLINCYTO permanently.
	Grade 4	Consider discontinuing BLINCYTO permanently.

* Based on the Common Terminology Criteria for Adverse Events (CTCAE). Grade 3 is severe, and Grade 4 is life-threatening.

Preparation

It is very important that the instructions for preparation (including admixing) and administration provided in this section are strictly followed to minimize medication errors (including underdose and overdose) [see Warnings and Precautions]

BLINCYTO can be infused over 24 hours (preservative-free) or 48 hours (preservative-free), or 7 days (with preservative). The choice between these options for the infusion duration should be made by the treating physician considering the frequency of the infusion bag changes and the weight of the patient. The 7-day infusion is not recommended for patients weighing less than 22 kg.

For preparation, reconstitution, and administration of BLINCYTO:

See Section 2.5 for infusion over 24 hours or 48 hours.

See Section 2.6 for infusion over 7 days using Bacteriostatic 0.9% Sodium Chloride Injection, USP (containing 0.9% benzyl alcohol). This option is available for patients weighing greater than or equal to 22 kg. It is not recommended for patients weighing less than 22 kg.

Call 1-800-77-AMGEN (1-800-772-6436) if you have questions about the reconstitution and preparation of BLINCYTO.

Aseptic Preparation

Strictly observe aseptic technique when preparing the solution for infusion since BLINCYTO vials do not contain antimicrobial preservatives. To prevent accidental contamination, prepare BLINCYTO according to aseptic standards, including but not limited to:

Prepare BLINCYTO in a USP <797> compliant facility.

Prepare BLINCYTO in an ISO Class 5 laminar flow hood or better.

Ensure that the admixing area has appropriate environmental specifications, confirmed by periodic monitoring.

Ensure that personnel are appropriately trained in aseptic manipulations and admixing of oncology drugs.

Ensure that personnel wear appropriate protective clothing and gloves.

Ensure that gloves and surfaces are disinfected.

Package Content

1 package BLINCYTO includes 1 vial of BLINCYTO and 1 vial of IV Solution Stabilizer.

Do not use IV Solution Stabilizer for reconstitution of BLINCYTO. IV Solution Stabilizer is provided with the BLINCYTO package and is used to coat the IV bag prior to addition of reconstituted BLINCYTO to prevent adhesion of BLINCYTO to IV bags and IV tubing.

More than 1 package of BLINCYTO may be needed to prepare some of the prescribed doses.

Aseptic Preparation

Strictly observe aseptic technique when preparing the solution for infusion since BLINCYTO vials do not contain antimicrobial preservatives. To prevent accidental contamination, prepare BLINCYTO according to aseptic standards, including but not limited to:

Prepare BLINCYTO in a USP <797> compliant facility.

Prepare BLINCYTO in an ISO Class 5 laminar flow hood or better.

Ensure that the admixing area has appropriate environmental specifications, confirmed by periodic monitoring.

Ensure that personnel are appropriately trained in aseptic manipulations and admixing of oncology drugs.

Ensure that personnel wear appropriate protective clothing and gloves.

Ensure that gloves and surfaces are disinfected.

Package Content

1 package BLINCYTO includes 1 vial of BLINCYTO and 1 vial of IV Solution Stabilizer.

Do not use IV Solution Stabilizer for reconstitution of BLINCYTO. IV Solution Stabilizer is provided with the BLINCYTO package and is used to coat the IV bag prior to addition of reconstituted BLINCYTO to prevent adhesion of BLINCYTO to IV bags and IV tubing.

More than 1 package of BLINCYTO may be needed to prepare some of the prescribed doses.

Incompatibility Information

BLINCYTO is incompatible with di-ethylhexylphthalate (DEHP) due to the possibility of particle formation, leading to a cloudy solution.

Use polyolefin, PVC DEHP-free, or ethyl vinyl acetate (EVA) infusion bags/pump cassettes. Use polyolefin, PVC DEHP-free, or EVA IV tubing sets.

8.1. Use 24-Hour or 48-Hour Infusion of BLINCYTO

8.1.1. Preparation of BLINCYTO Infusion Bag for 24- or 48-Hour Infusion

Verify the prescribed dose and infusion duration for each BLINCYTO infusion bag. To minimize errors, **use the specific volumes described in Tables 4 to 6 to prepare the BLINCYTO infusion bag.**

Table 4 for patients weighing greater than or equal to 45 kg

Tables 5 and 6 for patients weighing less than 45 kg

1. **Aseptically add 270 mL 0.9% Sodium Chloride Injection, USP to the IV bag.**
2. **Aseptically transfer 5.5 mL IV Solution Stabilizer** to the IV bag containing 0.9% Sodium Chloride Injection, USP. Gently mix the contents of the bag to avoid foaming. Discard the vial containing the unused IV Solution Stabilizer.
3. Aseptically transfer reconstituted BLINCYTO [see Dosage and Administration (2.5.2)] into the IV bag containing 0.9% Sodium Chloride Injection, USP and IV Solution Stabilizer. Gently mix the contents of the bag to avoid foaming.

Refer to Tables 4 to 6 for the specific volume of reconstituted BLINCYTO.

4. Under aseptic conditions, attach the IV tubing to the IV bag with the sterile 0.2 micron in-line filter.

Ensure that the IV tubing is compatible with the infusion pump.

5. Remove air from the IV bag. This is particularly important for use with an ambulatory infusion pump. **Prime the IV tubing only with the prepared solution for infusion. Do not prime with 0.9% Sodium Chloride Injection, USP.**
6. Store at 2°C to 8°C if not used immediately [see Dosage and Administration (2.7)].

Table 4. For Patients Weighing Greater Than or Equal to 45 kg: Volumes to Add to IV Bag

0.9% Sodium Chloride Injection, USP (starting volume)			270 mL
IV Solution Stabilizer			5.5 mL
Dose	Infusion Duration	Infusion Rate	Reconstituted BLINCYTO
9 mcg/day	24 hours	10 mL/hour	0.83 mL
	48 hours	5 mL/hour	1.7 mL
28 mcg/day	24 hours	10 mL/hour	2.6 mL
	48 hours	5 mL/hour	5.2 mL*

* 2 packages of BLINCYTO are needed for preparation of 28 mcg/day dose infused over 48 hours at a rate of 5 mL/hour.

Table 5. For Patients Weighing Less Than 45 kg: Volumes to Add to IV Bag for 5 mcg/m2/day Dose

0.9% Sodium Chloride Injection, USP (starting volume)				270 mL
IV Solution Stabilizer				5.5 mL
Dose	**Infusion Duration**	**Infusion Rate**	**BSA (m^2)**	**Reconstituted BLINCYTO**
			1.5 – 1.59	0.7 mL
			1.4 – 1.49	0.66 mL
			1.3 – 1.39	0.61 mL
			1.2 – 1.29	0.56 mL
			1.1 – 1.19	0.52 mL
5 $mcg/m^2/day$	24 hours	10 mL/hour	1 – 1.09	0.47 mL
			0.9 – 0.99	0.43 mL
			0.8 – 0.89	0.38 mL
			0.7 – 0.79	0.33 mL
			0.6 – 0.69	0.29 mL
			0.5 – 0.59	0.24 mL
			0.4 – 0.49	0.2 mL
			1.5 – 1.59	1.4 mL
			1.4 – 1.49	1.3 mL

5 mcg/m²/day	48 hours	5 mL/hour	1.3 – 1.39	1.2 mL
			1.2 – 1.29	1.1 mL
			1.1 – 1.19	1 mL
			1 – 1.09	0.94 mL
			0.9 – 0.99	0.85 mL
			0.8 – 0.89	0.76 mL
			0.7 – 0.79	0.67 mL
			0.6 – 0.69	0.57 mL
			0.5 – 0.59	0.48 mL
			0.4 – 0.49	0.39 mL

Table 6. For Patients Weighing Less Than 45 kg: Volumes to Add to IV Bag for 15 mcg/m²/day Dose

0.9% Sodium Chloride Injection, USP (starting volume)				270 mL
IV Solution Stabilizer				5.5 mL
Dose	**Infusion Duration**	**Infusion Rate**	**BSA (m²)**	**Reconstituted BLINCYTO**
			1.5 – 1.59	2.1 mL
			1.4 – 1.49	2 mL
			1.3 – 1.39	1.8 mL
			1.2 – 1.29	1.7 mL

			1.1 – 1.19	1.6 mL
15 mcg/m²/day	24 hours	10 mL/hour	1 – 1.09	1.4 mL
			0.9 – 0.99	1.3 mL
			0.8 – 0.89	1.1 mL
			0.7 – 0.79	1 mL
			0.6 – 0.69	0.86 mL
			0.5 – 0.59	0.72 mL
			0.4 – 0.49	0.59 mL
			1.5 – 1.59	4.2 mL*
			1.4 – 1.49	3.9 mL*
			1.3 – 1.39	3.7 mL*
			1.2 – 1.29	3.4 mL*
			1.1 – 1.19	3.1 mL*
15 mcg/m²/day	48 hours	5 mL/hour	1 – 1.09	2.8 mL
			0.9 – 0.99	2.6 mL
			0.8 – 0.89	2.3 mL
			0.7 – 0.79	2 mL
			0.6 – 0.69	1.7 mL
			0.5 – 0.59	1.4 mL
			0.4 – 0.49	1.2 mL

* 2 packages of BLINCYTO are needed for preparation of 15 mcg/m^2/day dose infused over 48 hours at a rate of 5 mL/hour for patients with a BSA greater than 1.09 m^2.

8.1.2. Reconstitution of BLINCYTO

1. Add 3 mL of preservative-free Sterile Water for Injection, USP by directing the water along the walls of the BLINCYTO vial and not directly on the lyophilized powder (resulting in a final BLINCYTO concentration of 12.5 mcg/mL).

Do not reconstitute BLINCYTO with IV Solution Stabilizer.

2. Gently swirl contents to avoid excess foaming. **Do not shake.**
3. Visually inspect the reconstituted solution for particulate matter and discoloration during reconstitution and prior to infusion. The resulting solution should be clear to slightly opalescent, colorless to slightly yellow. **Do not use if solution is cloudy or has precipitated.**

8.1.3. Administration

- Administer BLINCYTO as a continuous intravenous infusion at a constant flow rate using an infusion pump. The pump should be programmable, lockable, non-elastomeric, and have an alarm.
- Prepared BLINCYTO infusion bags [see Dosage and Administration (2.5.1)] should be infused over 24 hours or 48 hours.
- The starting volume (270 mL) is more than the volume administered to the patient (240 mL) to account for the priming of the IV tubing and to ensure that the patient will receive the full dose of BLINCYTO.
- Infuse BLINCYTO solution according to the instructions on the pharmacy label on the prepared bag at one of the following constant infusion rates:
- Infusion rate of 10 mL/hour for a duration of 24 hours, OR
- Infusion rate of 5 mL/hour for a duration of 48 hours
- The BLINCYTO solution must be administered using IV tubing that contains a sterile, non-pyrogenic, low protein-binding, 0.2 micron in-line filter.
- **Important Note: Do not flush the BLINCYTO infusion line or intravenous catheter, especially when changing infusion bags. Flushing when changing bags or at completion of infusion can result in excess dosage and complications thereof. When administering via a multi-lumen venous catheter, BLINCYTO should be infused through a dedicated lumen.**

- At the end of the infusion, any unused BLINCYTO solution in the IV bag and IV tubing should be disposed of in accordance with local requirements.

8.2. 7-Day Infusion of BLINCYTO using Bacteriostatic Saline

This option is not recommended for use in patients weighing less than 22 kg [see Warnings and Precautions (5.12) and Use in Specific Populations (8.4)].

8.2.1. Preparation of BLINCYTO Infusion Bag for 7-Day Infusion

Verify the prescribed dose and infusion duration for each BLINCYTO infusion bag. **To minimize errors, use the specific volumes described in Table 7 to prepare the BLINCYTO infusion bag.**

1. **Aseptically add 90 mL Bacteriostatic 0.9% Sodium Chloride Injection, USP to the empty IV bag.**
2. **Aseptically transfer 2.2 mL IV Solution Stabilizer to the IV bag containing the saline solution.** Gently mix the contents of the bag to avoid foaming. Discard the vial containing the unused IV Solution Stabilizer.
3. **Aseptically transfer reconstituted BLINCYTO** [see Dosage and Administration (2.6.2)] into the IV bag containing the saline solution and IV Solution Stabilizer. Gently mix the contents of the bag to avoid foaming.
- Refer to Table 7 for the specific volume of reconstituted BLINCYTO.
4. **Aseptically add 0.9% Sodium Chloride Injection, USP to the IV bag to a final volume of**

110 mL resulting in 0.74% benzyl alcohol. Gently mix the contents of the bag to avoid foaming.

- Refer to Table 7 for the specific volume of 0.9% Sodium Chloride Injection, USP.
5. Under aseptic conditions, attach the IV tubing to the IV bag. An in-line filter is not required for a 7-day bag.
- Ensure that the IV tubing is compatible with the infusion pump.
6. Remove air from the IV bag. This is particularly important for use with an ambulatory infusion pump. **Prime the IV tubing only with the prepared solution for infusion. Do not prime with 0.9% Sodium Chloride Injection, USP.**

Store at 2°C to 8°C if not used immediately [see Dosage and Administration (2.7)].

Table 7. For 7-Day Infusion: Volumes to Add to IV Bag for 28 mcg/day and 15 mcg/m²/day; Not Recommended for Patients Less Than 22 kg

Bacteriostatic 0.9% Sodium Chloride Injection, USP (starting volume)	90 mL
IV Solution Stabilizer	2.2 mL
Reconstituted BLINCYTO	Specific volume listed below in table
Quantity Sufficient (qs) with 0.9% Sodium Chloride Injection, USP to a Final Volume of 110 mL	
Infusion Duration	7 days
Infusion Rate	0.6 mL/hour

Patient Weight	**Dose**	**BSA (m^2)**	**Number of BLINCYTO Packages**	**Reconstituted BLINCYTO**	**0.9% Sodium Chloride Injection, USP to qs to a Final Volume of 110 mL**
Greater than or equal to 45 kg (fixed-dose)	28 mcg/day		6	16.8 mL	1 mL

22-45 kg (BSA-based dose)	15 mcg/m²/day	1.5 – 1.59	5	14 mL	3.8 mL
		1.4 – 1.49	5	13.1 mL	4.7 mL
		1.30 – 1.39	5	12.2 mL	5.6 mL
		1.20 – 1.29	5	11.3 mL	6.5 mL
		1.10 – 1.19	4	10.4 mL	7.4 mL
		1 – 1.09	4	9.5 mL	8.3 mL
		0.9 – 0.99	4	8.6 mL	9.2 mL

8.2.2. Reconstitution of BLINCYTO

Add 3 mL of preservative-free Sterile Water for Injection, USP by directing the water along the walls of the BLINCYTO vial and not directly on the lyophilized powder (resulting in a final BLINCYTO concentration of 12.5 mcg/mL).

Do not reconstitute BLINCYTO with IV Solution Stabilizer.

Gently swirl contents to avoid excess foaming. **Do not shake.**

Visually inspect the reconstituted solution for particulate matter and discoloration during reconstitution and prior to infusion. The resulting solution should be clear to slightly opalescent, colorless to slightly yellow. Do not use if solution is cloudy or has precipitated.

8.2.3. Administration

- Administer BLINCYTO as a continuous intravenous infusion at a constant flow rate using an infusion pump. The pump should be programmable, lockable, non-elastomeric, and have an alarm.
- Prepared BLINCYTO infusion bags [see Dosage and Administration (2.6.1)] should be infused over 7 days.
- The final volume of infusion solution (110 mL) will be more than the volume administered to the patient (100 mL) to account for the priming of the IV tubing and to ensure that the patient will receive the full dose of BLINCYTO.
- Infuse BLINCYTO solution according to the instructions on the pharmacy label on the prepared bag at an infusion rate of 0.6 mL/hour for a duration of 7 days.
- **Important Note: Do not flush the BLINCYTO infusion line or intravenous catheter, especially when changing infusion bags. Flushing when changing bags or at completion of infusion can result in excess dosage and complications thereof. When administering via a multi-lumen venous catheter, BLINCYTO should be infused through a dedicated lumen.**
- At the end of the infusion, any unused BLINCYTO solution in the IV bag and IV tubing should be disposed of in accordance with local requirements.

8.3. Storage Requirements

The information in Table 8 indicates the storage time for the reconstituted BLINCYTO vial and prepared infusion bag.

Store lyophilized BLINCYTO and IV Solution Stabilizer vials for a maximum of 8 hours at room temperature in the original carton to protect from light [see How Supplied/Storage and Handling (16.2)].

Table 8. Storage Time for Reconstituted BLINCYTO Vial and Prepared BLINCYTO Infusion Bag

	Maximum Storage Time	
	Room Temperature 23°C to 27°C (73°F to 81°F)	Refrigerated 2°C to 8°C (36°F to 46°F)

Reconstituted BLINCYTO Vial	4 hours	24 hours
Prepared BLINCYTO Infusion Bag (Preservative-Free)	48 hours*	8 days
Prepared BLINCYTO Infusion Bag (with Preservative)	7 days*	14 days

* Storage time includes infusion time. If the prepared BLINCYTO infusion bag is not administered within the time frames and temperatures indicated, it must be discarded; it should not be refrigerated again.

9. DOSAGE FORMS AND STRENGTHS

For injection: 35 mcg of lyophilized powder in a single-dose vial for reconstitution.

10. CONTRAINDICATIONS

BLINCYTO is contraindicated in patients with known hypersensitivity to blinatumomab or to any component of the product formulation.

11. WARNINGS AND PRECAUTIONS

5.1. Cytokine Release Syndrome

Cytokine Release Syndrome (CRS), which may be life-threatening or fatal, occurred in patients receiving BLINCYTO. The median time to onset of CRS was 2 days after the start of infusion. Manifestations of CRS include fever, headache, nausea, asthenia, hypotension, increased alanine aminotransferase, increased aspartate aminotransferase, increased total bilirubin, and disseminated intravascular coagulation (DIC). The manifestations of CRS after treatment with BLINCYTO overlap with those of **infusion reactions, capillary leak syndrome (CLS), and hemophagocytic histiocytosis/macrophage activation syndrome (MAS).** Using all of these terms to define CRS in clinical trials of BLINCYTO, CRS was reported in 15% of patients with relapsed or refractory ALL and in 7% of patients with MRD-positive ALL.

Monitor patients for signs or symptoms of these events. Advise outpatients on BLINCYTO to contact their healthcare professional for signs and symptoms associated with CRS. If severe CRS occurs, interrupt

BLINCYTO until CRS resolves. Discontinue BLINCYTO permanently if life-threatening CRS occurs [see Dosage and Administration (2.3)].

5.2. Toxicities

In patients with ALL receiving BLINCYTO in clinical studies, neurological toxicities have occurred in approximately 65% of patients. Among patients that experienced a neurologic event, the median time to the first event was within the first 2 weeks of BLINCYTO treatment and the majority of events resolved. The most common (≥ 10%) manifestations of neurological toxicity were headache, and tremor; the neurological toxicity profile varied by age group [see Use in Specific Populations (8.4, 8.5)]. Grade 3 or higher (severe, life-threatening, or fatal) neurological toxicities following initiation of BLINCYTO administration occurred in approximately 13% of patients and included encephalopathy, convulsions, speech disorders, disturbances in consciousness, confusion and disorientation, and coordination and balance disorders. Manifestations of neurological toxicity included cranial nerve disorders. The majority of neurologic events resolved following interruption of BLINCYTO, but some resulted in treatment discontinuation.

There is limited experience with BLINCYTO in patients with active ALL in the central nervous system (CNS) or a history of neurologic events. Patients with a history or presence of clinically relevant CNS pathology were excluded from clinical studies.

Monitor patients receiving BLINCYTO for signs and symptoms of neurological toxicities. Advise outpatients on BLINCYTO to contact their healthcare professional if they develop signs or symptoms of neurological toxicities. Interrupt or discontinue BLINCYTO as recommended [see Dosage and Administration (2.3)].

5.3. Infections

In patients with ALL receiving BLINCYTO in clinical studies, serious infections such as sepsis, pneumonia, bacteremia, opportunistic infections, and catheter-site infections were observed in approximately 25% of patients, some of which were life-threatening or fatal. As appropriate, administer prophylactic antibiotics and employ surveillance testing during treatment with BLINCYTO. Monitor patients for signs and symptoms of infection and treat appropriately.

5.4. Tumor Lysis Syndrome *(and see Appendix X)*

Tumor lysis syndrome (TLS), which may be life-threatening or fatal, has been observed in patients receiving BLINCYTO. Appropriate prophylactic measures, including pretreatment nontoxic cytoreduction and on-treatment hydration, should be used for the prevention of TLS during BLINCYTO treatment. Monitor for signs or symptoms of TLS. Management of these events may require either temporary interruption or discontinuation of BLINCYTO [see Dosage and Administration (2.3)].

11.1. Neutropenia and Febrile Neutropenia

Neutropenia and febrile neutropenia, including life-threatening cases, have been observed in patients receiving BLINCYTO. Monitor laboratory parameters (including, but not limited to, white blood cell count and absolute neutrophil count) during BLINCYTO infusion. Interrupt BLINCYTO if prolonged neutropenia occurs.

11.2. Effects on Ability to Drive and Use Machines

Due to the potential for neurologic events, including seizures, patients receiving BLINCYTO are at risk for loss of consciousness [see Warnings and Precautions (5.2)]. Advise patients to refrain from driving and engaging in hazardous occupations or activities such as operating heavy or potentially dangerous machinery while BLINCYTO is being administered.

11.3. Elevated Liver Enzymes

Treatment with BLINCYTO was associated with transient elevations in liver enzymes. In patients with ALL receiving BLINCYTO in clinical studies, the median time to onset of elevated liver enzymes was 3 days.

The majority of these transient elevations in liver enzymes were observed in the setting of CRS. For the events that were observed outside the setting of CRS, the median time to onset was 19 days. Grade 3 or greater elevations in liver enzymes occurred in approximately 7% of patients outside the setting of CRS and resulted in treatment discontinuation in less than 1% of patients.

Monitor alanine aminotransferase (ALT), aspartate aminotransferase (AST), gamma-glutamyl transferase (GGT), and total blood bilirubin prior to the start of and during BLINCYTO treatment. Interrupt BLINCYTO if the transaminases rise to greater than 5 times the upper limit of normal or if total bilirubin rises to more than 3 times the upper limit of normal.

11.4. Pancreatitis

Fatal pancreatitis has been reported in patients receiving BLINCYTO in combination with dexamethasone in clinical studies and the postmarketing setting [see Adverse Reactions (6.2)].

Evaluate patients who develop signs and symptoms of pancreatitis. Management of pancreatitis may require either temporary interruption or discontinuation of BLINCYTO and dexamethasone [see Dosage and Administration (2.3)].

11.5. Leukoencephalopathy

Cranial magnetic resonance imaging (MRI) changes showing leukoencephalopathy have been observed in patients receiving BLINCYTO, especially in patients with prior treatment with cranial irradiation and antileukemic chemotherapy (including systemic high-dose methotrexate or intrathecal cytarabine). The clinical significance of these imaging changes is unknown.

11.6. Preparation and Administration Errors

Preparation and administration errors have occurred with BLINCYTO treatment. Follow instructions for preparation (including admixing) and administration strictly to minimize medication errors (including underdose and overdose) [see Dosage and Administration (2.4)].

11.7. Immunization

The safety of immunization with live viral vaccines during or following BLINCYTO therapy has not been studied. Vaccination with live virus vaccines is not recommended for at least 2 weeks prior to the start of BLINCYTO treatment, during treatment, and until immune recovery following last cycle of BLINCYTO.

11.8. Risk of Serious Adverse Reactions in Pediatric Patients due to Benzyl Alcohol Preservative

Serious and fatal adverse reactions including "gasping syndrome" can occur in neonates and infants treated with benzyl alcohol-preserved drugs, including BLINCYTO (with preservative). The "gasping syndrome" is characterized by central nervous system depression, metabolic acidosis, and gasping respirations.

When prescribing BLINCYTO (with preservative) for pediatric patients, consider the combined daily metabolic load of benzyl alcohol from all sources including BLINCYTO (with preservative) (contains 7.4 mg of benzyl alcohol per mL) and other drugs containing benzyl alcohol. The minimum amount of benzyl alcohol at which serious adverse reactions may occur is not known [see Use in Specific Populations (8.4)].

Due to the addition of bacteriostatic saline, 7-day bags of BLINCYTO solution for infusion with preservative contain benzyl alcohol and are not recommended for use in any patients weighing less than 22 kg [see Dosage and Administration (2.6) and Use in Specific Populations (8.4)].

12. ADVERSE REACTIONS

The following adverse reactions are discussed in greater detail in other sections of the label:

Cytokine Release Syndrome [see Warnings and Precautions (5.1)]

Neurological Toxicities [see Warnings and Precautions (5.2)]

Infections [see Warnings and Precautions (5.3)]

Tumor Lysis Syndrome [see Warnings and Precautions (5.4)]

Neutropenia and Febrile Neutropenia [see Warnings and Precautions (5.5)]

Effects on Ability to Drive and Use Machines [see Warnings and Precautions (5.6)]

Elevated Liver Enzymes [see Warnings and Precautions (5.7)]

Pancreatitis [see Warnings and Precautions (5.8)]

Leukoencephalopathy [see Warnings and Precautions (5.9)]

Clinical Trials Experience

Because clinical trials are conducted under widely varying conditions, adverse reaction rates observed in the clinical trials of a drug cannot be directly compared to rates in the clinical trials of another drug and may not reflect the rates observed in practice.

MRD-positive B-cell Precursor ALL

The safety of BLINCYTO in patients with MRD-positive B-cell precursor ALL was evaluated in two single-arm clinical studies in which 137 patients were treated with BLINCYTO. The median age of the study population was 45 years (range: 18 to 77 years).

The most common adverse reactions (≥ 20%) were pyrexia, infusion related reactions, headache, infections (pathogen unspecified), tremor, and chills. Serious adverse reactions were reported in 61% of patients. The most common serious adverse reactions (≥ 2%) included pyrexia, tremor, encephalopathy, aphasia, lymphopenia, neutropenia, overdose, device related infection, seizure, and staphylococcal infection. Adverse reactions of Grade 3 or higher were reported in 64% of patients. Discontinuation of therapy due to adverse reactions occurred in 17% of patients; neurologic events were the most frequently reported reasons for discontinuation. There were 2 fatal adverse events that occurred within 30 days of the end of BLINCYTO treatment (atypical pneumonia and subdural hemorrhage).

Table 9 summarizes the adverse reactions occurring at a ≥ 10% incidence for any grade or ≥ 5% incidence for Grade 3 or higher.

Table 9. Adverse Reactions Occurring at ≥ 10% Incidence for Any Grade or ≥ 5% Incidence for Grade 3 or Higher in BLINCYTO-Treated Patients with MRD-Positive B-cell Precursor ALL (N=137)

Adverse reaction	**Any grade*** **n %**	**Equal to, or greater than, Grade 3** **n %**
Blood and lymphatic system disorders		
Neutropenia[1]	21 (15)	21 (15)
Leukopenia[2]	19 (14)	13 (9)
Thrombocytopenia[3]	14 (10)	8 (6)
Cardiac disorders		
Arrythmia[4]	17 (12)	3 (2)
General disorders and administration site conditions		
Pyrexia[5]	125 (91)	9 (7)
Chills	39 (28)	0 (0)
Infections and infestations		
Infections – pathogen unspecified	53 (39)	11 (8)
Injury, poisoning and procedural complications		
Infusion-related reaction	105 (77)	7 (5)
Investigations		
Decreased immunoglobulins[7]	25 (18)	7 (5)
Weight increase	14 (10)	1 (<1)
Hypertransaminemia[8]	13 (9)	9 (7)

Musculo-skeletal and connective tissue disorder		
Back pain	16 (12)	1 (<1)
Nervous system disorders		
Headache	39 (54)	5 (4)
Tremor[9]	43 (31)	6(4)
Aphasia	16 (12)	1 (<1)
Dizziness	14 (10)	1 (<1)
Encephalopathy[10]	14 (10)	6(4)
Psychiatric disorders		
Insomnia[11]	24 (18)	1 (<1)
Respiratory, thoracic and mediastinal disorders		
Cough	18 (13)	0 (<0)
Skin and subcutaneous disorders		
Rash	22 (16)	1 (<1)
Vascular disorders		
Hypertension	19 (14)	1 (<1)

* Grading based on NCI Common Terminology for Adverse Events (CTCAE) version 4.0

[1] Neutropenia includes febrile neutropenia, neutropenia, and neutrophil count decreased

[2] Thrombocytopenia includes platelet count decreased and thrombocytopenia

[3] Leukopenia includes leukopenia and white blood cell count decreased

[4] Arrhythmia includes bradycardia, sinus arrhythmia, sinus bradycardia, sinus tachycardia, tachycardia and ventricular extrasystoles

[5] Pyrexia includes body temperature increased and pyrexia

[6] Infusion-related reaction is a composite term that includes the term infusion-related reaction and the following events occurring with the first 48 hours of infusion and the event lasted ≤ 2 days: cytokine release syndrome, eye swelling, hypertension, hypotension, myalgia, periorbital edema, pruritus generalized, pyrexia, and rash

[7] Decreased immunoglobulins includes blood immunoglobulin A decreased, blood immunoglobulin G decreased, blood immunoglobulin M decreased, hypogammaglobulinemia, hypoglobulinemia, and immunoglobulins decreased

[8] Hypertransaminasemia includes alanine aminotransferase increased, aspartate aminotransferase increased, and hepatic enzyme increased

[9] Tremor includes essential tremor, intention tremor, and tremor

[10] Encephalopathy includes cognitive disorder, depressed level of consciousness, disturbance in attention, encephalopathy, lethargy, leukoencephalopathy, memory impairment, somnolence, and toxic encephalopathy

[11] Insomnia includes initial insomnia, insomnia, and terminal insomnia

[12] Rash includes dermatitis contact, eczema, erythema, rash, and rash maculopapular

Table 9. Adverse Reactions Occurring at ≥ 10% Incidence for Any Grade or ≥ 5% Incidence for Grade 3 or Higher in BLINCYTO-Treated Patients with MRD-Positive B-cell Precursor ALL (N=137)

Adverse Reaction	Any Grade* n (%)	≥ Grade 3* n (%)
Hypertransaminasemia[8]	13 (9)	9 (7)
Musculoskeletal and connective tissue disorders		
Back pain	16 (12)	1 (<1)
Nervous system disorders		
Headache	54 (39)	5 (4)
Tremor[9]	43 (31)	6 (4)
Aphasia	16 (12)	1 (<1)
Dizziness	14 (10)	1 (<1)
Encephalopathy[10]	14 (10)	6 (4)
Psychiatric disorders		
Insomnia[11]	24 (18)	1 (<1)
Respiratory, thoracic and mediastinal disorders		
Cough	18 (13)	0 (0)
Skin and subcutaneous tissue disorders		
Rash[12]	22 (16)	1 (<1)
Vascular disorders		
Hypotension	19 (14)	1 (<1)

* Grading based on NCI Common Terminology for Adverse Events (CTCAE) version 4.0

[1] Neutropenia includes febrile neutropenia, neutropenia, and neutrophil count decreased

[2] Thrombocytopenia includes platelet count decreased and thrombocytopenia

[3] Leukopenia includes leukopenia and white blood cell count decreased

[4] Arrhythmia includes bradycardia, sinus arrhythmia, sinus bradycardia, sinus tachycardia, tachycardia and ventricular extrasystoles

[5] Pyrexia includes body temperature increased and pyrexia

[6] Infusion-related reaction is a composite term that includes the term infusion-related reaction and the following events occurring with the first 48 hours of infusion and the event lasted ≤ 2 days: cytokine release syndrome, eye swelling, hypertension, hypotension, myalgia, periorbital edema, pruritus generalized, pyrexia, and rash

[7] Decreased immunoglobulins includes blood immunoglobulin A decreased, blood immunoglobulin G decreased, blood immunoglobulin M decreased, hypogammaglobulinemia, hypoglobulinemia, and immunoglobulins decreased

[8] Hypertransaminasemia includes alanine aminotransferase increased, aspartate aminotransferase increased, and hepatic enzyme increased

[9] Tremor includes essential tremor, intention tremor, and tremor

[10] Encephalopathy includes cognitive disorder, depressed level of consciousness, disturbance in attention, encephalopathy, lethargy, leukoencephalopathy, memory impairment, somnolence, and toxic encephalopathy

[11] Insomnia includes initial insomnia, insomnia, and terminal insomnia

[12] Rash includes dermatitis contact, eczema, erythema, rash, and rash maculopapular

Additional adverse reactions in patients with MRD-positive ALL that did not meet the threshold criteria for inclusion in Table 9 were:

Blood and lymphatic system disorders: anemia

General disorders and administration site conditions: edema peripheral, pain, and chest pain (includes chest pain and musculoskeletal chest pain)

Hepatobiliary disorders: blood bilirubin increased

Immune system disorders: hypersensitivity and cytokine release syndrome

Infections and infestations: viral infectious disorders, bacterial infectious disorders, and fungal infectious disorders

Injury, poisoning and procedural complications: medication error and overdose (includes overdose and accidental overdose)

Investigations: blood alkaline phosphatase increased

Musculoskeletal and connective tissue disorders: pain in extremity and bone pain

Nervous system disorders: seizure (includes seizure and generalized tonic-clonic seizure), speech disorder, and hypoesthesia

Psychiatric disorders: confusional state, disorientation, and depression

Respiratory, thoracic and mediastinal disorders: dyspnea and productive cough

Vascular disorders: hypertension (includes blood pressure increased and hypertension) flushing (includes flushing and hot flush), and capillary leak syndrome

Philadelphia Chromosome-negative Relapsed or Refractory B-cell Precursor ALL

The safety data described below reflect exposure to BLINCYTO in a randomized, open-label, active-controlled clinical study (TOWER Study) in which 376 patients with Philadelphia chromosome-negative relapsed or refractory B-cell precursor ALL were treated with BLINCYTO (n = 267) or standard of care (SOC) chemotherapy (n = 109). The median age of BLINCYTO-treated patients was 37 years (range: 18 to 80 years), 60% were male, 84% were White, 7% Asian, 2% were Black or African American, 2% were American Indian or Alaska Native, and 5% were Multiple/Other.

The most common adverse reactions (≥ 20%) in the BLINCYTO arm were infections (bacterial and pathogen unspecified), pyrexia, headache, infusion-related reactions, anemia, febrile neutropenia, thrombocytopenia, and neutropenia. Serious adverse reactions were reported in 62% of patients. The most common serious adverse reactions (≥ 2%) included febrile neutropenia, pyrexia, sepsis, pneumonia, overdose, septic shock, CRS, bacterial sepsis, device related infection, and bacteremia. Adverse reactions of Grade 3 or higher were reported in 87% of patients. Discontinuation of therapy due to adverse reactions occurred in 12% of patients treated with BLINCYTO; neurologic events and infections were the most frequently reported reasons for discontinuation of treatment due to an adverse reaction. Fatal adverse events occurred in 16% of patients. The majority of the fatal events were infections.

The adverse reactions occurring at a ≥ 10% incidence for any grade or ≥ 5% incidence for Grade 3 or higher in the BLINCYTO-treated patients in first cycle of therapy are summarized in Table 10.

Table 10. Adverse Reactions Occurring at ≥ 10% Incidence for Any Grade or ≥ 5% Incidence for Grade 3 or Higher in BLINCYTO-treated Patients in First Cycle of Therapy

	BLINCYTO (N = 267)		**Standard of Care (SOC) Chemotherapy (N = 109)**	
Adverse Reaction	**Any Grade* n (%)**	**≥ Grade 3* n (%)**	**Any Grade* n (%)**	**≥ Grade 3* n (%)**
Blood and lymphatic system disorders				
Neutropenia[1]	84 (31)	76 (28)	67 (61)	61 (56)
Anemia[2]	68 (25)	52 (19)	45 (41)	37 (34)
Thrombocytopenia[3]	57 (21)	47 (18)	42 (39)	40 (37)
Leukopenia4	21 (8)	18 (7)	9 (8)	9 (8)
Cardiac disorders				
Arrhythmia[5]	37 (14)	5 (2)	18 (17)	0 (0)
General disorders and administration site conditions				

Pyrexia	147 (55)	15 (6)	43 (39)	4 (4)
Edema[6]	48 (18)	3 (1)	20 (18)	1 (1)
Immune system disorders				
Cytokine release syndrome[7]	37 (14)	8 (3)	0 (0)	0 (0)
Infections and infestations				
Infections - pathogen unspecified	74 (28)	40 (15)	50 (46)	35 (32)
Bacterial infectious disorders	38 (14)	19 (7)	35 (32)	21 (19)
Viral infectious disorders	30 (11)	4 (1)	14 (13)	0 (0)
Fungal infectious disorders	27 (10)	13 (5)	15 (14)	9 (8)
Injury, poisoning and procedural complications				
Infusion-related reaction[8]	79 (30)	9 (3)	9 (8)	1 (1)
Investigations				
Hypertransaminasemia[9]	40 (15)	22 (8)	13 (12)	7 (6)
Nervous system disorders				
Headache	61 (23)	1 (<1)	30 (28)	3 (3)
Skin and subcutaneous tissue disorders				
Rash[10]	31 (12)	2 (1)	21 (19)	0 (0)

*Grading based on NCI Common Terminology Criteria for Adverse Events (CTCAE) version 4.0

[1]Neutropenia includes agranulocytosis, febrile neutropenia, neutropenia, and neutrophil count decreased

[2]Anemia includes anemia and hemoglobin decreased

[3]Thrombocytopenia includes platelet count decreased and thrombocytopenia

[4]Leukopenia includes leukopenia and white blood cell count decreased

[5]Arrhythmia includes arrhythmia, atrial fibrillation, atrial flutter, bradycardia, sinus bradycardia, sinus tachycardia, supraventricular tachycardia, and tachycardia

[6]Edema includes face edema, fluid retention, edema, edema peripheral, peripheral swelling, and swelling face

[7]Cytokine release syndrome includes cytokine release syndrome and cytokine storm

[8]Infusion-related reaction is a composite term that includes the term infusion-related reaction and the following events occurring with the first 48 hours of infusion and the event lasted ≤ 2 days: pyrexia, cytokine release syndrome, hypotension, myalgia, acute kidney injury, hypertension, and rash erythematous

[9]Hypertransaminasemia includes alanine aminotransferase increased, aspartate aminotransferase increased, hepatic enzyme increased, and transaminases increased

[10]Rash includes erythema, rash, rash erythematous, rash generalized, rash macular, rash maculo-papular, rash pruritic, skin exfoliation, and toxic skin eruption.

Selected laboratory abnormalities worsening from baseline Grade 0-2 to treatment-related maximal Grade 3-4 in first cycle of therapy are shown in Table 11.

Table 11. Selected Laboratory Abnormalities Worsening from Baseline Grade 0-2 to Treatment-related Maximal Grade 3-4* in First Cycle of Therapy

	BLINCYTO **Grade 3 or 4 (%)**	**SOC Chemotherapy** **Grade 3 or 4 (%)**
Hematology		
Decreased lymphocyte count	80	83
Decreased white blood cell count	53	97
Decreased hemoglobin	29	43
Decreased neutrophil count	57	68
Decreased platelet count	47	85
Chemistry		
Increased ALT	11	11
Increased bilirubin	5	4
Increased AST	8	4

* Includes only patients who had both baseline and at least one laboratory measurement during first cycle of therapy available.

Relapsed or Refractory B-cell Precursor ALL

Other important adverse reactions from pooled relapsed or refractory B-cell precursor ALL studies were: **Blood and lymphatic system disorders**: lymphadenopathy, hematophagic histiocytosis, and leukocytosis (includes leukocytosis and white blood cell count increased)

General disorders and administration site conditions: chills, chest pain (includes chest discomfort, chest pain, musculoskeletal chest pain, and non-cardiac chest pain), pain, body temperature increased, hyperthermia, and systemic inflammatory response syndrome

Hepatobiliary disorders: hyperbilirubinemia (includes blood bilirubin increased and hyperbilirubinemia) Immune system disorders: hypersensitivity (includes hypersensitivity, anaphylactic reaction, angioedema, dermatitis allergic, drug eruption, drug hypersensitivity, erythema multiforme, and urticaria) Injury, poisoning and procedural complications: medication error and overdose (includes overdose, medication error, and accidental overdose)

Investigations: weight increased, decreased immunoglobulins (includes immunoglobulins decreased, blood immunoglobulin A decreased, blood immunoglobulin G decreased, blood immunoglobulin M decreased, and hypogammaglobulinemia), blood alkaline phosphatase increased, and hypertransaminasemia

Metabolism and nutrition disorders: tumor lysis syndrome

Musculoskeletal and connective tissue disorders: back pain, bone pain, and pain in extremity

Nervous system disorders: tremor (resting tremor, intention tremor, essential tremor, and tremor), altered state of consciousness (includes altered state of consciousness, depressed level of consciousness, disturbance in attention, lethargy, mental status changes, stupor, and somnolence), dizziness, memory impairment, seizure (includes seizure, and atonic seizure), aphasia, cognitive disorder, speech disorder, hypoesthesia, encephalopathy, and cranial nerve disorders (trigeminal neuralgia, trigeminal nerve disorder, sixth nerve paralysis, cranial nerve disorder, facial nerve disorder, and facial paresis).

Psychiatric disorders: insomnia, disorientation, confusional state, and depression (includes depressed mood, depression, suicidal ideation, and completed suicide)

Respiratory, thoracic and mediastinal disorders: dyspnea (includes acute respiratory failure, dyspnea, dyspnea exertional, respiratory failure, respiratory distress, bronchospasm, bronchial hyperreactivity, tachypnea, and wheezing), cough, and productive cough

Vascular disorders: hypotension (includes blood pressure decreased, hypotension, hypovolemic shock, and circulatory collapse), hypertension (includes blood pressure increased, hypertension, and hypertensive crisis), flushing (includes flushing and hot flush), and capillary leak syndrome

6.2. Postmarketing Experience

The following adverse reactions have been identified during postapproval use of BLINCYTO. Because these reactions are reported voluntarily from a population of uncertain size, it is not always possible to reliably estimate their frequency or establish a causal relationship to drug exposure.

Fatal pancreatitis has been reported in patients receiving BLINCYTO in combination with dexamethasone [see Warnings and Precautions (5.8)].

6.3. Immunogenicity

As with all therapeutic proteins, there is potential for immunogenicity. The immunogenicity of BLINCYTO has been evaluated using either an electrochemiluminescence detection technology (ECL) or an enzyme-linked immunosorbent assay (ELISA) screening immunoassay for the detection of binding anti-blinatumomab antibodies. For patients whose sera tested positive in the screening immunoassay, an in vitro biological assay was performed to detect neutralizing antibodies.

In clinical studies, less than 2% of patients treated with BLINCYTO tested positive for binding

anti-blinatumomab antibodies. Of patients who developed anti-blinatumomab antibodies, 7 out of 9 (78%) had in vitro neutralizing activity. Anti-blinatumomab antibody formation may affect pharmacokinetics of BLINCYTO.

If formation of anti-blinatumomab antibodies with a clinically significant effect is suspected, contact Amgen at 1-800-77-AMGEN (1-800-772-6436) to discuss antibody testing.

The detection of anti-blinatumomab antibody formation is highly dependent on the sensitivity and specificity of the assay. Additionally, the observed incidence of antibody (including neutralizing antibody) positivity in an assay may be influenced by several factors, including assay methodology, sample handling, timing of sample collection, concomitant medications, and underlying disease. For these reasons, comparison of the incidence of antibodies to blinatumomab with the incidence of antibodies to other products may be misleading.

7. DRUG INTERACTIONS

No formal drug interaction studies have been conducted with BLINCYTO. Initiation of BLINCYTO treatment causes transient release of cytokines that may suppress CYP450 enzymes. The highest drug-drug interaction risk is during the first 9 days of the first cycle and the first 2 days of the second cycle in patients who are receiving concomitant CYP450 substrates, particularly those with a narrow therapeutic index. In these patients, monitor for toxicity (eg, warfarin) or drug concentrations (eg, cyclosporine). Adjust the dose of the concomitant drug as needed [see Clinical Pharmacology (12.2, 12.3)].

8. USE IN SPECIFIC POPULATIONS

8.1. Pregnancy

Risk Summary

Based on its mechanism of action, BLINCYTO may cause fetal harm including B-cell lymphocytopenia when administered to a pregnant woman [see Clinical Pharmacology (12.1)]. There are no data on the use of BLINCYTO in pregnant women. In animal reproduction studies, a murine surrogate molecule administered to pregnant mice crossed the placental barrier (see Data). Advise pregnant women of the potential risk to a fetus.

The background rate of major birth defects and miscarriage is unknown for the indicated population. In the U.S. general population, the estimated background risk of major birth defects and miscarriage in clinically recognized pregnancies is 2-4% and 15-20%, respectively.

Clinical Considerations

Fetal/Neonatal Adverse Reactions

Due to the potential for B-cell lymphocytopenia in infants following exposure to BLINCYTO in-utero, the infant's B lymphocytes should be monitored before the initiation of live virus vaccination [see Warnings and Precautions (5.11)].

Data

Animal Data

Animal reproduction studies have not been conducted with blinatumomab. In embryo-fetal developmental toxicity studies, a murine surrogate molecule was administered intravenously to pregnant mice during the period of organogenesis. The surrogate molecule crossed the placental barrier and did not cause embryo-fetal toxicity or teratogenicity. The expected depletions of B and T cells were observed in the pregnant mice, but hematological effects were not assessed in fetuses.

8.2. Lactation

Risk Summary

There is no information regarding the presence of blinatumomab in human milk, the effects on the breastfed infant, or the effects on milk production. Because many drugs are excreted in human milk and because of the potential for serious adverse reactions in nursing infants from BLINCYTO, including B-cell lymphocytopenia, advise patients not to breastfeed during and for at least 48 hours after treatment with BLINCYTO.

8.3. Females and Males of Reproductive Potential

Based on its mechanism of action, BLINCYTO may cause fetal harm when administered to a pregnant woman [see Use in Specific Populations (8.1)].

Pregnancy Testing

Verify the pregnancy status of females of reproductive potential prior to initiating BLINCYTO treatment.

Contraception

Females

Advise females of reproductive potential to use effective contraception during treatment and for at least 4 hours after the last dose of BLINCYTO.

8.4. Pediatric Use

The safety and efficacy of BLINCYTO have been established in pediatric patients with relapsed or refractory B-cell precursor ALL. Use of BLINCYTO is supported by a single-arm trial in pediatric patients with relapsed or refractory B-cell precursor ALL. This study included pediatric patients in the following age groups: 10 infants (1 month up to less than 2 years), 40 children (2 years up to less than 12 years), and 20 adolescents (12 years to less than 18 years). No differences in efficacy were observed between the different age subgroups. The efficacy has also been established based on extrapolation from adequate and well-controlled studies in adults with MRD-positive B-cell precursor ALL.

In general, the adverse reactions in BLINCYTO-treated pediatric patients were similar in type to those seen in adult patients with relapsed or refractory B-cell precursor ALL [see Adverse Reactions (6.1)]. Adverse reactions that were observed more frequently (≥ 10% difference) in the pediatric population compared to the adult population were pyrexia (80% vs. 61%), hypertension (26% vs. 8%), anemia (41% vs. 24%), infusion-related reaction (49% vs. 34%), thrombocytopenia (34% vs. 21%), leukopenia (24%

vs. 11%), and weight increased (17% vs. 6%).

In pediatric patients less than 2 years old (infants), the incidence of neurologic toxicities was not significantly different than for the other age groups, but its manifestations were different; the only event terms reported were agitation, headache, insomnia, somnolence, and irritability. Infants also had an increased incidence of hypokalemia (50%) compared to other pediatric age cohorts (15-20%) or adults (17%).

The steady-state concentrations of blinatumomab were comparable in adult and pediatric patients at the equivalent dose levels based on BSA-based regimens.

Benzyl Alcohol Toxicity in Pediatric Patients

Serious adverse reactions including fatal reactions and the "gasping syndrome" occurred in premature neonates and infants in the neonatal intensive care unit who received drugs containing benzyl alcohol as

a preservative. In these cases, benzyl alcohol dosages of 99 to 234 mg/kg/day produced high levels of benzyl alcohol and its metabolites in the blood and urine (blood levels of benzyl alcohol were 0.61 to 1.378 mmol/L). Additional adverse reactions included gradual neurological deterioration, seizures, intracranial hemorrhage, hematologic abnormalities, skin breakdown, hepatic and renal failure, hypotension, bradycardia, and cardiovascular collapse. Preterm, low-birth weight infants may be more likely to develop these reactions because they may be less able to metabolize benzyl alcohol.

When prescribing BLINCYTO (with preservative) in pediatric patients, consider the combined daily metabolic load of benzyl alcohol from all sources including BLINCYTO (with preservative) (contains 7.4 mg of benzyl alcohol per mL) and other drugs containing benzyl alcohol. The minimum amount of

benzyl alcohol at which serious adverse reactions may occur is not known [see Warnings and Precautions (5.12)].

Due to the addition of bacteriostatic saline, 7-day bags of BLINCYTO solution for infusion contain benzyl alcohol and are not recommended for use in patients weighing less than 22 kg. Prepare

BLINCYTO solution for infusion with preservative-free saline (24- or 48-hour bags) for use in patients weighing less than 22 kg [see Dosage and Administration (2.5)].

8.5. Geriatric Use

Of the total number of patients with ALL treated in clinical studies of BLINCYTO approximately 12% were 65 and over, while 2% were 75 and older. No overall differences in safety or effectiveness were observed between these patients and younger patients, and other reported clinical experience has not identified differences in responses between the elderly and younger patients. However, elderly patients experienced a higher rate of serious infections and neurological toxicities, including cognitive disorder, encephalopathy, and confusion [see Warnings and Precautions (5.2, 5.3)].

10. OVERDOSAGE

Overdoses have been observed, including one adult patient who received 133-fold the recommended therapeutic dose of BLINCYTO delivered over a short duration.

In the dose evaluation phase of the Phase 1/2 study in pediatric and adolescent patients with relapsed or refractory B-cell precursor ALL, one patient experienced a fatal cardiac failure event in the setting of life-threatening cytokine release syndrome (CRS) at a 30 mcg/m^2/day (higher than the maximum tolerated/recommended) dose [see Warnings and Precautions (5.1) and Adverse Reactions (6)].

Overdoses resulted in adverse reactions, which were consistent with the reactions observed at the recommended therapeutic dose and included fever, tremors, and headache. In the event of overdose, interrupt the infusion, monitor the patient for signs of toxicity, and provide supportive care [see Warnings and Precautions (5.10)]. Consider re-initiation of BLINCYTO at the correct therapeutic dose when all toxicities have resolved and no earlier than 12 hours after interruption of the infusion [see Dosage and Administration (2.1)].

17. DESCRIPTION

BLINCYTO (blinatumomab) is a bispecific CD19-directed CD3 T-cell engager that binds to CD19 (expressed on cells of B-lineage origin) and CD3 (expressed on T cells). BLINCYTO is produced in Chinese hamster ovary cells. It consists of 504 amino acids and has a molecular weight of approximately 54 kilodaltons.

Each BLINCYTO package contains 1 vial BLINCYTO and 1 vial IV Solution Stabilizer.

BLINCYTO is supplied in a single-dose vial as a sterile, preservative-free, white to off-white lyophilized powder for intravenous administration. Each single-dose vial of BLINCYTO contains 35 mcg blinatumomab, citric acid monohydrate (3.35 mg), lysine hydrochloride (23.23 mg),

polysorbate 80 (0.64 mg), trehalose dihydrate (95.5 mg), and sodium hydroxide to adjust pH to 7.0. After reconstitution with 3 mL of preservative-free Sterile Water for Injection, USP, the resulting concentration is 12.5 mcg/mL blinatumomab.

IV Solution Stabilizer is supplied in a single-dose vial as a sterile, preservative-free, colorless to slightly yellow, clear solution. Each single-dose vial of IV Solution Stabilizer contains citric acid monohydrate (52.5 mg), lysine hydrochloride (2283.8 mg), polysorbate 80 (10 mg), sodium hydroxide to adjust pH to 7.0, and water for injection.

18. CLINICAL PHARMACOLOGY

12.1. Mechanism of Action

Blinatumomab is a bispecific CD19-directed CD3 T-cell engager that binds to CD19 expressed on the surface of cells of B-lineage origin and CD3 expressed on the surface of T cells. It activates endogenous T cells by connecting CD3 in the T-cell receptor (TCR) complex with CD19 on benign and malignant

B cells. Blinatumomab mediates the formation of a synapse between the T-cell and the tumor cell, upregulation of cell adhesion molecules, production of cytolytic proteins, release of inflammatory cytokines, and proliferation of T cells, which result in redirected lysis of CD19+ cells.

12.2. Pharmacodynamics

During the continuous intravenous infusion over 4 weeks, the pharmacodynamic response was characterized by T-cell activation and initial redistribution, reduction in peripheral B cells, and transient cytokine elevation.

Peripheral T-cell redistribution (ie, T-cell adhesion to blood vessel endothelium and/or transmigration into tissue) occurred after start of BLINCYTO infusion or dose escalation. T-cell counts initially declined within 1 to 2 days and then returned to baseline levels within 7 to 14 days in the majority of patients.

Increase of T-cell counts above baseline (T-cell expansion) was observed in few patients.

Peripheral B cell counts decreased to less than or equal to 10 cells/microliter during the first treatment cycle at doses ≥ 5 mcg/m2/day or ≥ 9 mcg/day in the majority of patients. No recovery of peripheral B-cell counts was observed during the 2-week BLINCYTO-free period between treatment cycles.

Incomplete depletion of B cells occurred at doses of 0.5 mcg/m2/day and 1.5 mcg/m2/day and in a few patients at higher doses.

Cytokines including IL-2, IL-4, IL-6, IL-8, IL-10, IL-12, TNF-α, and IFN-γ were measured, and IL-6, IL-10, and IFN-γ were elevated. The highest elevation of cytokines was observed in the first 2 days following start of BLINCYTO infusion. The elevated cytokine levels returned to baseline within 24 to 48 hours during the infusion. In subsequent treatment cycles, cytokine elevation occurred in fewer patients with lesser intensity compared to the initial 48 hours of the first treatment cycle.

12.3. Pharmacokinetics

The pharmacokinetics of blinatumomab appear linear over a dose range from 5 to 90 mcg/m2/day (approximately equivalent to 9 to 162 mcg/day) in adult patients. Following continuous intravenous infusion, the steady-state serum concentration (Css) was achieved within a day and remained stable over time. The increase in mean Css values was approximately proportional to the dose in the range tested. At the clinical doses of 9 mcg/day and 28 mcg/day for the treatment of relapsed or refractory ALL, the mean (SD) Css was 228 (356) pg/mL and 616 (537) pg/mL, respectively.

Distribution

The estimated mean (SD) volume of distribution based on terminal phase (Vz) was 4.35 (2.45) L with continuous intravenous infusion of blinatumomab.

Metabolism

The metabolic pathway of blinatumomab has not been characterized. Like other protein therapeutics, BLINCYTO is expected to be degraded into small peptides and amino acids via catabolic pathways.

Elimination

The estimated mean (SD) systemic clearance with continuous intravenous infusion in patients receiving blinatumomab in clinical studies was 3.11 (2.98) L/hour. The mean (SD) half-life was 2.10 (1.41) hours. Negligible amounts of blinatumomab were excreted in the urine at the tested clinical doses.

Gender, Age, and Body Surface Area

Results of population pharmacokinetic analyses indicate that age (0.62 to 80 years of age) and gender do not influence the pharmacokinetics of blinatumomab. Body surface area (0.4 to 2.70 m2) influences the pharmacokinetics of blinatumomab, however, the clinical relevance of this effect is unknown.

Hepatic Impairment

No formal pharmacokinetic studies using BLINCYTO have been conducted in patients with hepatic impairment.

Renal Impairment

No formal pharmacokinetic studies of blinatumomab have been conducted in patients with renal impairment.

Pharmacokinetic analyses showed an approximately 2-fold difference in mean blinatumomab clearance values between patients with moderate renal impairment (CrCL ranging from 30 to 59 mL/min, N = 21) and normal renal function (CrCL more than 90 mL/min, N = 215). However, high interpatient variability was discerned (CV% up to 96.8%), and clearance values in renal impaired patients were essentially within the range observed in patients with normal renal function. There is no information available in patients with severe renal impairment (CrCL less than 30 mL/min) or patients on hemodialysis.

Drug Interactions

Transient elevation of cytokines may suppress CYP450 enzyme activities [see Drug Interactions (7) and Clinical Pharmacology (12.2)].

Specific Populations

Pediatrics: The pharmacokinetics of blinatumomab appear linear over a dose range from 5 to 30 mcg/m^2/day in pediatric patients. At the recommended doses, the mean (SD) steady-state concentration (Css) values were 162 (179) and 533 (392) pg/mL at 5 and 15 mcg/m^2/day doses,

respectively. The estimated mean (SD) volume of distribution (Vz), clearance (CL), and terminal half-life (t1/2,z) were 3.14 (2.97) L/m^2, 1.88 (1.90) L/hour/m^2, and 2.04 (1.35) hours, respectively.

19. CLINICAL TOXICOLOGY

13.1. Carcinogenesis, Mutagenesis, Impairment of Fertility

No carcinogenicity or genotoxicity studies have been conducted with blinatumomab.

No studies have been conducted to evaluate the effects of blinatumomab on fertility. A murine surrogate molecule had no adverse effects on male and female reproductive organs in a 13-week repeat-dose toxicity study in mice.

20. CLINICAL STUDIES

14.2. MRD-positive B-cell Precursor ALL

BLAST Study

The efficacy of BLINCYTO was evaluated in an open-label, multicenter, single-arm study (BLAST Study) [NCT01207388] that included patients who were ≥ 18 years of age, had received at least 3 chemotherapy blocks of standard ALL therapy, were in hematologic complete remission (defined as < 5% blasts in bone marrow, absolute neutrophil count > 1 Gi/L, platelets > 100 Gi/L) and had MRD at a level of ≥ 0.1% using an assay with a minimum sensitivity of 0.01%. BLINCYTO was administered at a constant dose of 15 mcg/m^2/day (equivalent to the recommended dosage of 28 mcg/day) intravenously for all treatment cycles. Patients received up to 4 cycles of treatment. Dose adjustment was possible in case of adverse events.

The treated population included 86 patients in first or second hematologic complete remission (CR1 or CR2). The demographics and baseline characteristics are shown in Table 12. The median number of treatment cycles was 2 (range: 1 to 4). Following treatment with BLINCYTO, 45 out of 61 (73.8%) patients in CR1 and 14 out of 25 (56.0%) patients in CR2 underwent allogeneic hematopoietic stem cell transplantation in continuous hematologic complete remission.

Table 12: Demographics and Baseline Characteristics in BLAST Study

Characteristic	**BLINCYTO (N = 86)**
Age	
Median, years (min, max)	43 (18,76)

≥ 65 years, n (%)	10 (12)
Males, n (%)	50 (58)
Race, n (%)	
Asian	1 (1)
Other (mixed)	0 (0)
White	76 (88)
Unknown	9 (11)
Philadelphia chromosome disease status, n (%)	
Positive	1 (1)
Negative	85 (99)
Relapse history, n (%)	
Patients in 1st CR	61 (71)
Patients in 2nd CR	25 (29)

Table 12: Demographics and Baseline Characteristics in BLAST Study

Characteristic	**BLINCYTO (N = 86)**
MRD level at baseline*, n (%)	
≥ 10%	7 (8)
≥ 1% and < 10%	34 (40)
≥ 0.1% and < 1%	45 (52)

* Assessed centrally using an assay with minimum sensitivity of 0.01%

Efficacy was based on achievement of undetectable MRD within one cycle of BLINCYTO treatment and hematological relapse-free survival (RFS). The assay used to assess MRD response had a sensitivity of 0.01% for 6 patients and < 0.005% for 80 patients. Overall, undetectable MRD was achieved by 70 patients (81.4%: 95% CI: 71.6%, 89.0%). The median hematological RFS was 22.3 months. Table 13 shows the MRD response and hematological RFS by remission number.

Table 13. Efficacy Results in Patients ≥ 18 Years of Age With MRD-positive B-cell Precursor ALL (BLAST Study)

	Patients in CR1 (n=61)	Patients in CR2 (n=25)
Complete MRD response[1], n (%), [95% CI]	52 (85.2) [73.8, 93.0]	18 (72.0) [50.6, 87.9]
Median hematological relapse-free survival[2] in months (range)	35.2 (0.4, 53.5)	12.3 (0.7, 42.3)

1. Complete MRD response was defined as the absence of detectable MRD confirmed in an assay with minimum sensitivity of 0.01%

2. Relapse was defined as either hematological or extramedullary relapse, secondary leukemia, or death due to any cause; Includes time after transplantation; Kaplan Meier estimate

Undetectable MRD was achieved by 65 of 80 patients (81.3%: 95% CI: 71.0%, 89.1%) with an assay sensitivity of at least 0.005%. The estimated median hematological RFS among the 80 patients using the higher sensitivity assay was 24.2 months (95% CI: 17.9, NE).

14.2. Relapsed/Refractory B-cell Precursor ALL

TOWER Study

The efficacy of BLINCYTO was compared to standard of care (SOC) chemotherapy in a randomized, open-label, multicenter study (TOWER Study) [NCT02013167]. Eligible patients were ≥ 18 years of age with relapsed or refractory B-cell precursor ALL [> 5% blasts in the bone marrow and refractory to primary induction therapy or refractory to last therapy, untreated first relapse with first remission duration

< 12 months, untreated second or later relapse, or relapse at any time after allogeneic hematopoietic stem cell transplantation (alloHSCT)]. BLINCYTO was administered at 9 mcg/day on Days 1-7 and

28 mcg/day on Days 8-28 for Cycle 1, and 28 mcg/day on Days 1-28 for Cycles 2-5 in 42-day cycles and for Cycles 6-9 in 84-day cycles. Dose adjustment was possible in case of adverse events. SOC chemotherapy included fludarabine, cytarabine arabinoside, and granulocyte colony-stimulating factor (FLAG); high-dose cytarabine arabinoside (HiDAC); high-dose methotrexate- (HDMTX) based combination; or clofarabine/clofarabine-based regimens.

There were 405 patients randomized 2:1 to receive BLINCYTO or investigator-selected SOC chemotherapy. Randomization was stratified by age (< 35 years vs. ≥ 35 years of age), prior salvage therapy (yes vs. no), and prior alloHSCT (yes vs. no) as assessed at the time of consent. The demographics and baseline characteristics were well-balanced between the two arms (see Table 14).

Table 14. Demographics and Baseline Characteristics in TOWER Study

Characteristic	**BLINCYTO (N = 271)**	**Standard of Care (SOC) Chemotherapy (N = 134)**
Age		
Median, years (min, max)	37 (18, 80)	37 (18, 78)
< 35 years, n (%)	124 (46)	60 (45)
≥ 35 years, n (%)	147 (54)	74 (55)
≥ 65 years, n (%)	33 (12)	15 (11)
≥ 75 years, n (%)	10 (4)	2 (2)
Males, n (%)	162 (60)	77 (58)
Race, n (%)		
American Indian or Alaska Native	4 (2)	1 (1)
Asian	19 (7)	9 (7)

Black (or African American)	5 (2)	3 (2)
Multiple	2 (1)	0
Native Hawaiian or Other Pacific Islander	1 (0)	1 (1)
Other	12 (4)	8 (6)
White	228 (84)	112 (84)
Prior salvage therapy	171 (63)	70 (52)
Prior alloHSCT[1]	94 (35)	46 (34)
Eastern Cooperative Group Status – n (%)		
0	96 (35)	52 (39)
1	134 (49)	61 (46)
2	41 (15)	20 (15)
Unknown	0	1 (1)
Refractory to salvage treatment - n (%)		
Yes	87 (32)	34 (25)
No	182 (67)	99 (74)
Unknown	2 (1)	1 (1)
Maximum of central/local bone marrow blasts - n (%)		
≤ 5%	0	0
> 5 to < 10%	9 (3)	7 (5)

10 to < 50%	60 (22)	23 (17)
≥ 50%	201 (74)	104 (78)
Unknown	1 (0)	0

[1]alloHSCT = allogeneic hematopoietic stem cell transplantation

Of the 271 patients randomized to the BLINCYTO arm, 267 patients received BLINCYTO treatment. The median number of treatment cycles was two (range: 1 to 9 cycles); 267 (99%) received Cycles 1-2 (induction), 86 (32%) received Cycles 3-5 (consolidation), and 27 (10%) received Cycles 6-9 (continued therapy). Of the 134 patients on the SOC arm, 25 dropped out prior to start of study treatment, and 109 patients received a median of 1 treatment cycle (range: 1 to 4 cycles).

The determination of efficacy was based on overall survival (OS). The study demonstrated statistically significant improvement in OS for patients treated with BLINCYTO as compared to SOC chemotherapy. See Figure 1 and Table 15 below for efficacy results from the TOWER Study.

Figure 1. Kaplan-Meier Curve of Overall Survival in TOWER Study

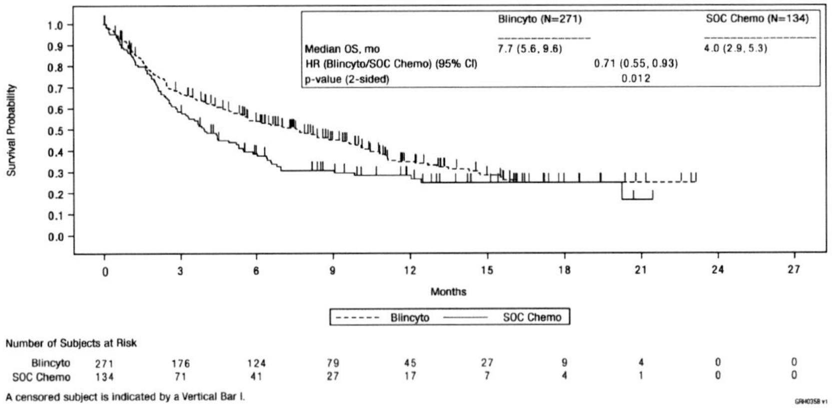

Table 15. Efficacy Results in Patients ≥ 18 Years of Age With Philadelphia Chromosome-Negative Relapsed or Refractory B-cell Precursor ALL (TOWER Study)

	BLINCYTO **(N = 271)**	**SOC Chemotherapy** **(N = 134)**
Overall Survival		
Number of deaths (%)	164 (61)	87 (65)
Median, months [95% CI]	7.7 [5.6, 9.6]	4.0 [2.9, 5.3]
Hazard Ratio [95% CI][1]	0.71 [0.55, 0.93]	
p-value[2]	0.012	
Overall Response		
CR[4]/CRh*[5], n (%) [95% CI]	115 (42) [37, 49]	27 (20) [14, 28]
Treatment difference [95% CI]	22 [13, 31]	
p-value[3]	< 0.001	
CR, n (%) [95% CI]	91 (34) [28, 40]	21 (16) [10, 23]
Treatment difference [95% CI]	18 [10, 26]	
p-value[3]	< 0.001	
MRD Response6 for CR/CRh*		
n1/n2 (%)[7] [95% CI]	73/115 (64) [54, 72]	14/27 (52) [32, 71]

[1]Based on stratified Cox's model.

[2]The p-value was derived using stratified log rank test.

[3]The p-value was derived using Cochran-Mantel-Haenszel test.

[4]CR (complete remission) was defined as ≤ 5% blasts in the bone marrow, no evidence of disease, and full recovery of peripheral blood counts (platelets > 100,000/microliter and absolute neutrophil counts [ANC] > 1,000/microliter).

[5]CRh* (complete remission with partial hematologic recovery) was defined as ≤ 5% blasts in the bone marrow, no evidence of disease, and partial recovery of peripheral blood counts (platelets > 50,000/microliter and ANC > 500/microliter).

[6]MRD (minimum residual disease) response was defined as MRD by PCR or flow cytometry < 1 x 10-4 (0.01%).

[7]n1: number of patients who achieved MRD response and CR/CRh*; n2: number of patients who achieved CR/CRh* and had a postbaseline assessment.

Study MT103-211

Study MT103-211 [NCT01466179] was an open-label, multicenter, single-arm study. Eligible patients were ≥ 18 years of age with Philadelphia chromosome-negative relapsed or refractory B-cell precursor ALL (relapsed with first remission duration of ≤ 12 months in first salvage or relapsed or refractory after first salvage therapy or relapsed within 12 months of alloHSCT, and had ≥ 10% blasts in bone marrow).

BLINCYTO was administered as a continuous intravenous infusion. The recommended dose for this study was determined to be 9 mcg/day on Days 1-7 and 28 mcg/day on Days 8-28 for Cycle 1, and

28 mcg/day on Days 1-28 for subsequent cycles. Dose adjustment was possible in case of adverse events. The treated population included 185 patients who received at least 1 infusion of BLINCYTO; the median number of treatment cycles was 2 (range: 1 to 5). Patients who responded to BLINCYTO but later relapsed had the option to be retreated with BLINCYTO. Among treated patients, the median age was 39 years (range: 18 to 79 years), 63 out of 185 (34.1%) had undergone HSCT prior to receiving BLINCYTO, and 32 out of 185 (17.3%) had received more than 2 prior salvage therapies.

Efficacy was based on the complete remission (CR) rate, duration of CR, and proportion of patients with an MRD-negative CR/CR with partial hematological recovery (CR/CRh*) within 2 cycles of treatment with BLINCYTO. Table 16 shows the efficacy results from this study. The HSCT rate among those who achieved CR/CRh* was 39% (30 out of 77).

Table 16. Efficacy Results in Patients ≥ 18 Years of Age With Philadelphia Chromosome-Negative Relapsed or Refractory B-cell Precursor ALL (Study MT103-211)

	N = 185		
	CR[1]	**CRh*[2]**	**CR/CRh***
n (%) [95% CI]	60 (32.4) [25.7 – 39.7]	17 (9.2) [5.4 – 14.3]	77 (41.6) [34.4 – 49.1]
MRD response[3]			
n1/n2 (%)[4] [95% CI]	48/60 (80.0) [67.7 – 89.2]	10/17 (58.8) [32.9 – 81.6]	58/77 (75.3) [64.2 – 84.4]
DOR/RFS[5]			
Median (months) (range)	6.7 (0.46 – 16.5)	5.0 (0.13 – 8.8)	5.9 (0.13 – 16.5)

[1]CR (complete remission) was defined as ≤ 5% of blasts in the bone marrow, no evidence of disease, and full recovery of peripheral blood counts (platelets > 100,000/microliter and absolute neutrophil counts [ANC] > 1,000/microliter).

[2]CRh* (complete remission with partial hematological recovery) was defined as ≤ 5% of blasts in the bone marrow, no evidence of disease, and partial recovery of peripheral blood counts (platelets > 50,000/microliter and ANC > 500/microliter).

[3]MRD (minimal residual disease) response was defined as MRD by PCR < 1 x 10-4 (0.01%).

[4]n1: number of patients who achieved MRD response and the respective remission status; n2: number of patients who achieved the respective remission status. Six CR/CRh* responders with missing MRD data were considered as MRD-nonresponders.

[5]DOR (duration of response)/RFS (relapse-free survival) was defined as time since first response of CR or CRh* to relapse or death, whichever is earlier. Relapse was defined as hematological relapse (blasts in bone marrow greater than 5% following CR) or an extramedullary relapse.

ALCANTARA Study

The efficacy of BLINCYTO for treatment of Philadelphia chromosome-positive B-cell precursor ALL was evaluated in an open-label, multicenter, single-arm study (ALCANTARA Study) [NCT02000427]. Eligible patients were ≥ 18 years of age with Philadelphia chromosome-positive B-cell precursor ALL, relapsed or refractory to at least 1 second generation or later tyrosine kinase inhibitor (TKI), or intolerant to second generation TKI, and intolerant or refractory to imatinib mesylate.

BLINCYTO was administered at 9 mcg/day on Days 1-7 and 28 mcg/day on Days 8-28 for Cycle 1, and 28 mcg/day on Days 1-28 for subsequent cycles. Dose adjustment was possible in case of adverse events.

The treated population included 45 patients who received at least one infusion of BLINCYTO; the median number of treatment cycles was 2 (range: 1 to 5). The demographics and baseline characteristics are shown in Table 17.

Table 17. Demographics and Baseline Characteristics in ALCANTARA Study

Characteristic	BLINCYTO (N = 45)
Age	
Median, years (min, max)	55 (23, 78)
≥ 65 years and < 75 years, n (%)	10 (22)
≥ 75 years, n (%)	2 (4)
Males, n (%)	24 (53)
Race, n (%)	
Asian	1 (2)
Black (or African American)	3 (7)
Other	2 (4)
White	39 (87)
Disease History	
Prior TKI treatment1, n (%)	
1	7 (16)
2	21 (47)
≥ 3	17 (38)
Prior salvage therapy	31 (62)
Prior alloHSCT2	20 (44)
Bone marrow blasts3	
≥ 50% to < 75%	6 (13)
≥ 75%	28 (62)

1 Number of patients that failed ponatinib = 23 (51%)

2 alloHSCT = allogeneic hematopoietic stem cell transplantation

3 centrally assessed

Efficacy was based on the complete remission (CR) rate, duration of CR, and proportion of patients with an MRD-negative CR/CR with partial hematological recovery (CR/CRh*) within 2 cycles of treatment with BLINCYTO. Table 18 shows the efficacy results from ALCANTARA Study. Five of the 16 responding (31%) patients underwent allogeneic HSCT in CR/CRh* induced with BLINCYTO. There were 10 patients with document T315I mutation; four achieved CR within 2 cycles of treatment with BLINCYTO.

Table 18. Efficacy Results in Patients ≥ 18 Years of Age With Philadelphia Chromosome-Positive Relapsed or Refractory B-cell Precursor ALL (ALCANTARA Study)

	N = 45		
	CR1	CRh*2	CR/CRh*
n (%) [95% CI]	14 (31) [18 – 47]	2 (4) [1 – 15]	16 (36) [22 – 51]
MRD response3			
n1/n2 (%)4 [95% CI]	12/14 (86) [57 – 98]	2/2 (100) [16, 100]	14/16 (88) [62 – 98]
DOR/RFS5			
Median (months) (range)	6.7 (3.6 – 12.0)	NE6 (3.7 – 9.0)	6.7 (3.6 – 12.0)

1 CR (complete remission) was defined as ≤ 5% of blasts in the bone marrow, no evidence of disease, and full recovery of peripheral blood counts (platelets > 100,000/microliter and absolute neutrophil counts [ANC] > 1,000/microliter).

2 alloHSCT = allogeneic hematopoietic stem cell transplantation

3 centrally assessed

Efficacy was based on the complete remission (CR) rate, duration of CR, and proportion of patients with an MRD-negative CR/CR with partial hematological recovery (CR/CRh*) within 2 cycles of treatment with BLINCYTO. Table 18 shows the efficacy results from ALCANTARA Study. Five of the 16 responding (31%) patients underwent allogeneic HSCT in CR/CRh* induced with BLINCYTO. There were 10 patients with document T315I mutation; four achieved CR within 2 cycles of treatment with BLINCYTO.

Table 18. Efficacy Results in Patients ≥ 18 Years of Age With Philadelphia Chromosome-Positive Relapsed or Refractory B-cell Precursor ALL (ALCANTARA Study)

	N = 45		
	CR1	CRh*2	CR/CRh*
n (%) [95% CI]	14 (31) [18 – 47]	2 (4) [1 – 15]	16 (36) [22 – 51]
MRD response3			
n1/n2 (%)4 [95% CI]	12/14 (86) [57 – 98]	2/2 (100) [16, 100]	14/16 (88) [62 – 98]
DOR/RFS5			
Median (months) (range)	6.7 (3.6 – 12.0)	NE6 (3.7 – 9.0)	6.7 (3.6 – 12.0)

1 CR (complete remission) was defined as ≤ 5% of blasts in the bone marrow, no evidence of disease, and full recovery of peripheral blood counts (platelets > 100,000/microliter and absolute neutrophil counts [ANC] > 1,000/microliter).

2 CRh* (complete remission with partial hematological recovery) was defined as ≤ 5% of blasts in the bone marrow, no evidence of disease, and partial recovery of peripheral blood counts (platelets > 50,000/microliter and

ANC > 500/microliter).

3 MRD (minimal residual disease) response was defined as MRD by PCR < 1 x 10-4 (0.01%).

4 n1: number of patients who achieved MRD response and the respective remission status; n2: number of patients who achieved the respective remission status. Six CR/CRh* responders with missing MRD data were considered as MRD-nonresponders.

5 DOR (duration of response)/RFS (relapse-free survival) was defined as time since first response of CR or CRh* to relapse or death, whichever is earlier. Relapse was defined as hematological relapse (blasts in bone marrow greater than 5% following CR) or an extramedullary relapse.

6 NE = not estimable

Study MT103-205

Study MT103-205 [NCT01471782] was an open-label, multicenter, single-arm study in pediatric patients with relapsed or refractory B-cell precursor ALL (second or later bone marrow relapse, any marrow relapse after allogeneic HSCT, or refractory to other treatments, and had > 25% blasts in bone marrow). BLINCYTO was administered at 5 mcg/m2/day on Days 1-7 and 15 mcg/m2/day on Days 8-28 for

Cycle 1, and 15 mcg/m2/day on Days 1-28 for subsequent cycles. Dose adjustment was possible in case of adverse events. Patients who responded to BLINCYTO but later relapsed had the option to be retreated with BLINCYTO.

Among the 70 treated patients, the median age was 8 years (range: 7 months to 17 years), 40 out of 70 (57.1%) had undergone allogeneic HSCT prior to receiving BLINCYTO, and 39 out of 70 (55.7%) had refractory disease. The median number of treatment cycles was 1 (range: 1 to 5).

Twenty-three out of 70 (32.9%) patients achieved CR/CRh* within the first 2 treatment cycles with

17 out of 23 (73.9%) occurring within Cycle 1 of treatment. See Table 19 for the efficacy results from the study. The HSCT rate among those who achieved CR/CRh* was 48%.

11. BESPONSA (inotuzumab ozogamicin) for injection, for intravenous use. Initial U.S. Approval 2017

WARNING: HEPATOTOXICITY, INCLUDING HEPATIC VENO-OCCLUSIVE DISEASE (VOD) (ALSO KNOWN AS SINUSOIDAL OBSTRUCTION SYNDROME and INCREASED RISK OF POST-HEMATOPOIETIC STEM CELL TRANSPLANT (HSCT) NON-RELAPSE MORTALITY

HEPATOTOXICITY, INCLUDING VOD

Hepatotoxicity, including fatal and life-threatening VOD occurred in patients with relapsed or refractory acute lymphoblastic leukemia (ALL) who received BESPONSA. The risk of VOD was greater in patients who underwent HSCT after BESPONSA treatment; use of HSCT conditioning regimens containing 2 alkylating agents and last total bilirubin

level ≥ upper limit of normal (ULN) before HSCT were significantly associated with an increased risk of VOD.

Other risk factors for VOD in patients treated with BESPONSA included ongoing or prior liver disease, prior HSCT, increased age, later salvage lines, and a greater number of BESPONSA treatment cycles.

Elevation of liver tests may require dosing interruption, dose reduction, or permanent discontinuation of BESPONSA. Permanently discontinue treatment if VOD occurs. If severe VOD occurs, treat according to standard medical practice [see Dosage and Administration (2.3) and Warnings and Precautions (5.1)].

INCREASED RISK OF POST-HSCT NON-RELAPSE MORTALITY

There was higher post-HSCT non-relapse mortality rate in patients receiving BESPONSA, resulting in a higher Day 100 post-HSCT mortality rate [see Warnings and Precautions (5.2)].

Mechanism of Action

Inotuzumab ozogamicin is a CD22-directed antibody-drug conjugate (ADC). Inotuzumab recognizes human CD22. The small molecule, N-acetyl-gamma-calicheamicin, is a cytotoxic agent that is covalently attached to the antibody via a linker. Nonclinical data suggest that the anticancer activity of inotuzumab ozogamicin is due to the binding of the ADC to CD22-expressing tumor cells, followed by internalization of the ADC-CD22 complex, and the intracellular release of N-acetyl-gamma-calicheamicin dimethylhydrazide via hydrolytic cleavage of the linker. Activation of N-acetyl-gamma-calicheamicin dimethylhydrazide induces double-strand DNA breaks, subsequently inducing cell cycle arrest and apoptotic cell death.

1. **INDICATIONS AND USAGE**

BESPONSA is indicated for the treatment of adults with **relapsed or refractory B-cell precursor acute lymphoblastic leukemia (ALL).**

2. **DOSAGE AND ADMINISTRATION**

2.1. Recommended Dosage

- Pre-medicate before each dose [see Dosage and Administration (2.2)].
- For the first cycle, the recommended total dose of BESPONSA for all patients is 1.8 mg/m^2 per cycle, administered as 3 divided doses on Day 1 (0.8 mg/m^2), Day 8 (0.5 mg/m^2), and Day 15 (0.5 mg/m^2). Cycle 1 is 3 weeks in duration, but may be extended to 4 weeks if the patient achieves a complete remission (CR) or complete remission with incomplete hematologic recovery (CRi), and/or to allow recovery from toxicity.
- For subsequent cycles:
- In patients who achieve a CR or CRi, the recommended total dose of BESPONSA is 1.5 mg/m^2 per cycle, administered as 3 divided doses on Day 1 (0.5 mg/m2), Day 8 (0.5 mg/m^2), and
- Day 15 (0.5 mg/m^2). Subsequent cycles are 4 weeks in duration.
  OR
- In patients who do not achieve a CR or CRi, the recommended total dose of BESPONSA is
- 1.8 mg/m^2 per cycle given as 3 divided doses on Day 1 (0.8 mg/m^2), Day 8 (0.5 mg/m^2), and Day 15 (0.5 mg/m^2). Subsequent cycles are 4 weeks in duration. Patients who do not achieve a CR or CRi within 3 cycles should discontinue treatment.

For patients proceeding to hematopoietic stem cell transplant (HSCT), the recommended duration of treatment with BESPONSA is 2 cycles. A third cycle may be considered for those

- patients who do not achieve CR or CRi and minimal residual disease (MRD) negativity after 2 cycles [see Warnings and Precautions (5.1)].
- For patients not proceeding to HSCT, additional cycles of treatment, up to a maximum of 6 cycles, may be administered.

Table 1 shows the recommended dosing regimens.

Table 1. Dosing Regimen for Cycle 1 and Subsequent Cycles Depending on Response to Treatment

	Day 1	**Day 8[a]**	**Day 15[a]**
Dosing regimen for Cycle 1			
All patients:			
Dose[b]	0.8 mg/m^2	0.5 mg/m^2	0.5 mg/m^2
Cycle length	21 days[c]		
Dosing regimen for subsequent cycles depending on response to treatment			
Patients who have achieved a CR[d] or CR1:[e]			
Doseb	0.5 mg/m^2	0.5 mg/m^2	0.5 mg/m^2
Cycle length	28 days[f]		
Patients who have not achieved a CR[d] or CR1[e]			
Dose[b]	0.8 mg/m^2	0.5 mg/m^2	0.5 mg/m^2
Cycle length	28 days[f]		

Abbreviations: CR=complete remission; CRi=complete remission with incomplete hematologic recovery.

[a] +/- 2 days (maintain minimum of 6 days between doses).

[b] Dose is based on the patient's body surface area (m^2).

[c] For patients who achieve a CR or a CRi, and/or to allow for recovery from toxicity, the cycle length may be extended up to 28 days (i.e., 7-day treatment-free interval starting on Day 21).

[d] CR is defined as < 5% blasts in the bone marrow and the absence of peripheral blood leukemic blasts, full recovery of peripheral blood counts (platelets ≥ 100 × 10^9/L and absolute neutrophil counts [ANC] ≥ 1 × 10^9/L) and resolution of any extramedullary disease.

[e] CRi is defined as < 5% blasts in the bone marrow and the absence of peripheral blood leukemic blasts, incomplete recovery of peripheral blood counts (platelets < 100 × 10^9/L and/or ANC < 1 × 10^9/L) and resolution of any extramedullary disease.

[f] 7-day treatment-free interval starting on Day

2.2. Recommended Pre-medications and Cytoreduction

- Premedication with a corticosteroid, antipyretic, and antihistamine is recommended prior to dosing. Patients should be observed during and for at least 1 hour after the end of infusion for symptoms of infusion related reactions [see Warnings and Precautions (5.4)].
- For patients with circulating lymphoblasts, cytoreduction with a combination of hydroxyurea, steroids, and/or vincristine to a peripheral blast count of less than or equal to 10,000/mm3 is recommended prior to the first dose.

2.3. Dose Modification

Modify the dose of BESPONSA for toxicities (see Tables 2-4). BESPONSA doses within a treatment cycle (i.e., Days 8 and/or 15) do not need to be interrupted due to neutropenia or thrombocytopenia, but dosing interruptions within a cycle are recommended for non-hematologic toxicities. If the dose is reduced due to BESPONSA-related toxicity, the dose must not be re-escalated.

Table 2. BESPONSA Dose Modifications for Hematologic Toxicities

Criteria	BESPONSA Dose Modification(s)
If prior to BESPONSA treatment ANC was greater than or equal to 1 × 10^9/L	If ANC decreases, then interrupt the next cycle of treatment until recovery of ANC to greater than or equal to 1 × 10^9/L. Discontinue BESPONSA if low ANC persists for greater than 28 days and is suspected to be related to BESPONSA.

If prior to BESPONSA treatment platelet count was greater than or equal to 50 × 10^9/L[a]	If platelet count decreases, then interrupt the next cycle of treatment until platelet count recovers to greater than or equal to 50 × 10^9/L[a]. Discontinue BESPONSA if low platelet count persists for greater than 28 days and is suspected to be related to BESPONSA.

If prior to BESPONSA treatment ANC was less than 1 × 10^9/L and/or platelet count was less than 50 × 10^9/L[a]	If ANC or platelet count decreases, then interrupt the next cycle of treatment until at least one of the following occurs: ANC and platelet counts recover to at least baseline levels for the prior cycle, or ANC recovers to greater than or equal to 1 × 10^9/L and platelet count recovers to greater than or equal to 50 × 10^9/L[a], or Stable or improved disease (based on most recent bone marrow assessment) and the ANC and platelet count decrease is considered to be due to the underlying disease (not considered to be BESPONSA-related toxicity).

Abbreviation: ANC=absolute neutrophil count.

[a] Platelet count used for dosing should be independent of blood transfusion.

Table 3. BESPONSA Dose Modifications for Non-hematologic Toxicities

Non-hematologic Toxicity	Dose Modification(s)
VOD or other severe liver toxicity	Permanently discontinue treatment [see Warnings and Precautions (5.1)].

Total bilirubin greater than 1.5 × ULN and AST/ALT greater than 2.5 × ULN	Interrupt dosing until recovery of total bilirubin to less than or equal to 1.5 × ULN and AST/ALT to less than or equal to 2.5 × ULN prior to each dose unless due to Gilbert's syndrome or hemolysis. Permanently discontinue treatment if total bilirubin does not recover to less than or equal to 1.5 × ULN or AST/ALT does not recover to less than or equal to 2.5 × ULN [see Warnings and Precautions (5.1)].
Infusion-related reaction	Interrupt the infusion and institute appropriate medical management. Depending on the severity of the infusion-related reaction, consider discontinuation of the infusion or administration of steroids and antihistamines. For severe or life-threatening infusion reactions, permanently discontinue treatment [see Warnings and Precautions (5.4)].
Non-hematologic toxicity greater than or equal to Grade 2[a]	Interrupt treatment until recovery to Grade 1 or pre-treatment grade levels prior to each dose.

Abbreviations: ALT=alanine aminotransferase; AST=aspartate aminotransferase; ULN=upper limit of normal; VOD=venoocclusive disease.

[a] Severity grade according to National Cancer Institute Common Terminology Criteria for Adverse Events (NCI CTCAE) version 3.0.

Table 4. BESPONSA Dose Modifications Depending on Duration of Dosing Interruption Due to Non-Hematologic Toxicity Toxicities

Duration of Dose Interruption Due to Toxicity	**Dose Modification(s)**
Less than 7 days (within a	Interrupt the next dose (maintain a minimum of 6 days between

cycle)	doses).
Greater than or equal to 7 days	Omit the next dose within the cycle.
Greater than or equal to 14 days	Once adequate recovery is achieved, decrease the total dose by 25% for the subsequent cycle. If further dose modification is required, then reduce the number of doses to 2 per cycle for subsequent cycles. If a 25% decrease in the total dose followed by a decrease to 2 doses per cycle is not tolerated, then permanently discontinue treatment.
Greater than 28 days	Consider permanent discontinuation of treatment.

2.5. Instructions for Reconstitution, Dilution, and Administration

Protect the reconstituted and diluted BESPONSA solutions from light. Do not freeze the reconstituted or diluted solution.

The maximum time from reconstitution through the end of administration should be less than or equal to 8 hours, with less than or equal to 4 hours between reconstitution and dilution.

Reconstitution

- BESPONSA is a cytotoxic drug. Follow applicable special handling and disposal procedures.
- Calculate the dose (mg) and number of vials of BESPONSA required.
- Reconstitute each vial with 4 mL of Sterile Water for Injection, USP, to obtain a concentration of

0.25 mg/mL of BESPONSA that delivers 3.6 mL (0.9 mg).

- Gently swirl the vial to aid dissolution. **DO NOT SHAKE.**
- Inspect the reconstituted solution for particulates and discoloration. The reconstituted solution should be clear to opalescent, colorless to slightly yellow, and essentially free of visible foreign matter.
- See Table 5 for storage times and conditions for the reconstituted solution.

Dilution

- Calculate the required volume of the reconstituted solution needed to obtain the appropriate dose according to the patient's body surface area. Withdraw this amount from the vial(s) using a syringe. Discard any unused reconstituted BESPONSA solution left in the vial.
- Add reconstituted solution to an infusion container with 0.9% Sodium Chloride Injection, USP, to a make a total volume of 50 mL. An infusion container made of polyvinyl chloride (PVC)

(di(2-ethylhexyl)phthalate [DEHP]- or non-DEHP-containing), polyolefin (polypropylene and/or polyethylene), or ethylene vinyl acetate (EVA) is recommended.

- Gently invert the infusion container to mix the diluted solution. **DO NOT SHAKE**.
- See Table 5 for storage times and conditions for the diluted solution.

Administration

- See Table 5 for storage times and conditions for prior to and during administration of the diluted solution.
- Filtration of the diluted solution is not required. However, if the diluted solution is filtered, polyethersulfone (PES)-, polyvinylidene fluoride (PVDF)-,or hydrophilic polysulfone (HPS)-based filters are recommended. Do not use filters made of nylon or mixed cellulose ester (MCE).
- Infuse the diluted solution for 1 hour at a rate of 50 mL/h at room temperature (20-25°C; 68-77°F). Infusion lines made of PVC (DEHP- or non-DEHP-containing), polyolefin (polypropylene and/or polyethylene), or polybutadiene are recommended.
- Do not mix BESPONSA or administer as an infusion with other medicinal products.

Table 5 shows the storage times and conditions for reconstitution, dilution, and administration of BESPONSA.

Table 5. Storage Times and Conditions for Reconstituted and Diluted BESPONSA Solution

Maximum time from reconstitution through end of administration less than or equal to 8 hours[a]		
	Diluted Solution	
Reconstituted Solution	**After Start of Dilution**	**Administration**

BESPONSA contains no bacteriostatic preservatives. Use reconstituted solution immediately or after being refrigerated (2-8°C; 36-46°F) for up to 4 hours. **PROTECT FROM LIGHT. DO NOT FREEZE.**	Use diluted solution immediately or after storage at room temperature (20-25°C; 68-77°F) for up to 4 hours or being refrigerated (2-8°C; 36-46°F) for up to 3 hours. **PROTECT FROM LIGHT. DO NOT FREEZE**.	If the diluted solution is refrigerated (2-8°C; 36-46°F), allow it to equilibrate at room temperature (20-25°C; 68-77°F) for approximately 1 hour prior to administration. Administer diluted solution within 8 hours of reconstitution as a 1-hour infusion at a rate of 50 mL/h at room temperature (20-25°C; 68-77°F). **PROTECT FROM LIGHT.**

[a] With less than or equal to 4 hours between reconstitution and dilution.

3. DOSAGE FORMS AND STRENGTHS

For Injection: 0.9 mg as a white to off-white lyophilized powder in a single-dose vial for reconstitution and further dilution.

4. CONTRAINDICATIONS

None.

5. WARNINGS AND PRECAUTIONS

Hepatotoxicity, Including Hepatic Veno-occlusive Disease (VOD) (also known as Sinusoidal Obstruction Syndrome)

In the INO-VATE ALL trial, hepatotoxicity, including severe, life-threatening, and sometimes fatal hepatic VOD was observed in 23/164 patients (14%) in the BESPONSA arm during or following treatment or following a HSCT after completion of treatment. VOD was reported up to 56 days after the last dose during treatment or during follow-up without an intervening HSCT. The median time from subsequent HSCT to onset of VOD was 15 days (range: 3-57 days). In the BESPONSA arm, among the 79 patients who proceeded to a subsequent HSCT, VOD was reported in 18/79 patients (23%), and among all 164 patients treated, VOD was reported in 5/164 patients (3%) during study therapy or in follow-up without an intervening HSCT.

The risk of VOD was greater in patients who underwent HSCT after BESPONSA treatment; use of HSCT conditioning regimens containing 2 alkylating agents (e.g., busulfan in combination with other alkylating agents) and last total bilirubin level greater than or equal to the ULN before HSCT are significantly associated with an increased risk of VOD. Other risk factors for VOD in patients treated with BESPONSA included ongoing or prior liver disease, prior HSCT, increased age, later salvage lines, and a greater number of BESPONSA treatment cycles. Patients who have experienced prior VOD or have serious ongoing hepatic liver disease (e.g., cirrhosis, nodular regenerative hyperplasia, active hepatitis) are at an increased risk for worsening of liver disease, including developing VOD, following treatment with BESPONSA.

Monitor closely for signs and symptoms of VOD; these may include elevations in total bilirubin, hepatomegaly (which may be painful), rapid weight gain, and ascites. Due to the risk of VOD, for patients proceeding to HSCT, the recommended duration of treatment with BESPONSA is 2 cycles; a third cycle may be considered for those patients who do not achieve a CR or CRi and MRD negativity after 2 cycles [see Dosage and Administration (2.1)]. For patients who proceed to HSCT, monitor liver tests closely during the first month post-HSCT, then less frequently thereafter, according to standard medical practice.

(The most important histopathological characteristics of sinusoidal obstruction syndrome(SOS) are:

1. *Sinusoidal dilation*
2. *Portal tract changes of fibrosis and bile ductular reaction*
3. *Sclerosis of venular walls*
4. *Sinusoidal endothelial cell detachment from the space of Disse can be seen on electron microscopy*

Clinically SOS (VOD) is characterised by weight gain due to fluid retention, increased liver size, and raised levels of bilirubin in the blood).

In the INO-VATE ALL trial, increases in liver tests were reported. Grade 3/4 AST, ALT, and total bilirubin abnormal liver tests occurred in 7/160 (4%), 7/161 (4%), and 8/161 patients (5%), respectively.

In all patients, monitor liver tests, including ALT, AST, total bilirubin, and alkaline phosphatase, prior to and following each dose of BESPONSA. Elevations of liver tests may require dosing interruption, dose reduction, or permanent discontinuation of BESPONSA [see Dosage and Administration (2.3)].

5.2. Increased Risk of Post-Transplant Non-Relapse Mortality

In the INO-VATE ALL trial, a higher post-HSCT non-relapse mortality rate was observed in patients receiving BESPONSA compared to the Investigator's choice of chemotherapy arm, resulting in a higher Day 100 post-HSCT mortality rate.

Overall, 79/164 patients (48%) in the BESPONSA arm and 35/162 patients (22%) in the Investigator's choice of chemotherapy arm had a follow-up HSCT. The post-HSCT non-relapse mortality rate was 31/79 (39%) and 8/35 (23%) in the BESPONSA arm compared to the Investigator's choice of chemotherapy arm, respectively.

In the BESPONSA arm, the most common causes of post-HSCT non-relapse mortality included VOD and infections. Five of the 18 VOD events that occurred post-HSCT were fatal. In the BESPONSA arm, among patients with ongoing VOD at time of death, 6 patients died due to multiorgan failure (MOF) or infection (3 patients died due to MOF, 2 patients died due to infection, and 1 patient died due to MOF and infection).

Monitor closely for toxicities post-HSCT, including signs and symptoms of infection and VOD [see Warnings and Precautions (5.1, 5.3)].

5.3. Myelosuppression

In the INO-VATE ALL trial, myelosuppression was observed in patients receiving BESPONSA [see Adverse Reactions (6.1)].

Thrombocytopenia and neutropenia were reported in 83/164 patients (51%) and 81/164 patients (49%), respectively. Grade 3 thrombocytopenia and neutropenia were reported in 23/164 patients (14%) and 33/164 patients (20%), respectively. Grade 4 thrombocytopenia and neutropenia were reported in 46/164 patients (28%) and 45/164 patients (27%), respectively. Febrile neutropenia, which may be life-threatening, was reported in 43/164 patients (26%). For patients who were in CR or CRi at the end of treatment, the recovery of platelet counts to > 50,000/mm^3 was later than 45 days after the last dose in15/164 patients (9%) who received BESPONSA and 3/162 patients (2%) who received Investigator's choice of chemotherapy.

Complications associated with myelosuppression (including infections and bleeding/hemorrhagic events) were observed in patients receiving BESPONSA [see Adverse Reactions (6.1)]. Infections, including serious infections, some of which were life-threatening or fatal, were reported in 79/164 patients (48%). Fatal infections, including pneumonia, neutropenic sepsis, sepsis, septic shock, and pseudomonal sepsis, were reported in 8/164 patients (5%). Bacterial, viral, and fungal infections were reported.

Hemorrhagic events were reported in 54/164 patients (33%). Grade 3 or 4 hemorrhagic events were reported in 8/164 patients (5%). One Grade 5 (fatal) hemorrhagic event (intra-abdominal hemorrhage) was reported in 1/164 patients (1%). The most common hemorrhagic event was epistaxis which was reported in 24/164 patients (15%).

Monitor complete blood counts prior to each dose of BESPONSA and monitor for signs and symptoms of infection, bleeding/hemorrhage, or other effects of myelosuppression during treatment with BESPONSA. As appropriate, administer prophylactic anti-infectives and employ surveillance testing during and after treatment with BESPONSA. Management of severe infection, bleeding/hemorrhage, or other effects of myelosuppression, including severe neutropenia or thrombocytopenia, may require dosing interruption, dose reduction, or permanent discontinuation of BESPONSA [see Dosage and Administration (2.3)].

5.4. Infusion-Related Reactions

In the INO-VATE ALL trial, infusion-related reactions were observed in patients who received BESPONSA. Infusion related reactions (all Grade 2) were reported in 4/164 patients (2%). Infusion related reactions generally occurred in Cycle 1 shortly after the end of the BESPONSA infusion and resolved spontaneously or with medical management.

Premedicate with a corticosteroid, antipyretic, and antihistamine prior to dosing [see Dosage and Administration (2.2)].

Monitor patients closely during and for at least 1 hour after the end of infusion for the potential onset of infusion related reactions, including symptoms such as fever, chills, rash, or breathing problems. Interrupt infusion and institute appropriate medical management if an infusion related reaction occurs. Depending on the severity of the infusion related reaction, consider discontinuation of the infusion or administration of steroids and antihistamines. For severe or life-threatening infusion reactions, permanently discontinue BESPONSA [see Dosage and Administration (2.3)].

5.5. QT Interval Prolongation

In the INO-VATE ALL trial, increases in QT interval corrected for heart rate using Fridericia's formula (QTcF) of ≥ to 60 msec from baseline were measured in 4/162 patients (3%). No patients had QTcF values greater than 500 msec [see Clinical Pharmacology (12.2)]. Grade 2 QT prolongation was reported in 2/164 patients (1%). No ≥ Grade 3 QT prolongation or events of Torsade de Pointes were reported [see Adverse Reactions (6.1)].

Administer BESPONSA with caution in patients who have a history of or predisposition for QTc prolongation, who are taking medicinal products that are known to prolong QT interval [see Drug Interactions (7)], and in patients with electrolyte disturbances [see Drug Interactions (7)]. Obtain

electrocardiograms (ECGs) and electrolytes prior to the start of treatment, after initiation of any drug known to prolong QTc, and periodically monitor as clinically indicated during treatment [see Drug Interactions (7), Clinical Pharmacology (12.2)]).

5.6. Embryo-Fetal Toxicity

Based on its mechanism of action and findings from animal studies, BESPONSA can cause embryo-fetal harm when administered to a pregnant woman. In animal studies, inotuzumab ozogamicin caused embryo-fetal toxicities, starting at a dose that was approximately 0.4 times the exposure in patients at the maximum recommended dose, based on the area under the concentration-time curve (AUC). Advise

females of reproductive potential to use effective contraception during treatment with BESPONSA and for at least 8 months after the final dose of BESPONSA. Advise males with female partners of reproductive potential to use effective contraception during treatment with BESPONSA and for at least 5 months after the last dose of BESPONSA. Apprise pregnant women of the potential risk to the fetus. Advise women to contact their healthcare provider if they become pregnant or if pregnancy is suspected during treatment with BESPONSA [see Use in Specific Populations (8.1, 8.3), Clinical Pharmacology (12.1), Nonclinical Toxicology (13.1)].

6. ADVERSE REACTIONS

The following adverse reactions are discussed in greater detail in other sections of the label:

Hepatotoxicity, including hepatic VOD (also known as SOS) [see Warnings and Precautions (5.1)]

Increased risk of post-transplant non-relapse mortality [see Warnings and Precautions (5.2)]

Myelosuppression [see Warnings and Precautions (5.3)]

Infusion related reactions [see Warnings and Precautions (5.4)]

QT interval prolongation [see Warnings and Precautions (5.5)]

6.1. Clinical Trials Experience

Because clinical trials are conducted under widely varying conditions, adverse reaction rates observed in the clinical trials of a drug cannot be directly compared to rates in the clinical trials of another drug and may not reflect the rates observed in practice.

The adverse reactions described in this section reflect exposure to BESPONSA in 164 patients with relapsed or refractory ALL who participated in a randomized clinical study of BESPONSA versus Investigator's choice of chemotherapy (fludarabine + cytarabine + granulocyte colony-stimulating factor [FLAG], mitoxantrone + cytarabine [MXN/Ara-C], or high dose cytarabine [HIDAC]) (INO-VATE ALL Trial [NCT01564784]) [see Clinical Studies (14)].

Of the 164 patients who received BESPONSA, the median age was 47 years (range: 18-78 years), 56% were male, 68% had received 1 prior treatment regimen for ALL, 31% had received 2 prior treatment regimens for ALL, 68% were White, 19% were Asian, and 2% were Black.

In patients who received BESPONSA, the median duration of treatment was 8.9 weeks

(range: 0.1-26.4 weeks), with a median of 3 treatment cycles started in each patient. In patients who

received Investigator's choice of chemotherapy, the median duration of treatment was 0.9 weeks (range: 0.1-15.6 weeks), with a median of 1 treatment cycle started in each patient.

In patients who received BESPONSA, the most common (≥ 20%) adverse reactions were thrombocytopenia, neutropenia, infection, anemia, leukopenia, fatigue, hemorrhage, pyrexia, nausea, headache, febrile neutropenia, transaminases increased, abdominal pain, gamma-glutamyltransferase increased, and hyperbilirubinemia.

In patients who received BESPONSA, the most common (≥ 2%) serious adverse reactions were infection, febrile neutropenia, hemorrhage, abdominal pain, pyrexia, VOD, and fatigue.

In patients who received BESPONSA, the most common (≥ 2%) adverse reactions reported as the reason for permanent discontinuation were infection (6%), thrombocytopenia (2%), hyperbilirubinemia (2%), transaminases increased (2%), and hemorrhage (2%); the most common (≥ 5%) adverse reactions reported as the reason for dosing interruption were neutropenia (17%), infection (10%), thrombocytopenia (10%), transaminases increased (6%), and febrile neutropenia (5%); and the most common (≥ 1%) adverse reactions reported as the reason for dose reduction were neutropenia (1%), thrombocytopenia (1%), and transaminases increased (1%).

VOD was reported in 23/164 patients (14%) who received BESPONSA during or following treatment or following a HSCT after completion of treatment [see Warnings and Precautions (5.1)].

Table 6 shows the adverse reactions with ≥ 10% incidence reported in patients with relapsed or refractory ALL who received BESPONSA or Investigator's choice of chemotherapy.

Table 6. Adverse Reactions With ≥ 10% Incidence[a] in Patients With Relapsed or Refractory B-Cell Precursor ALL Who Received BESPONSA or Investigator's Choice of Chemotherapy (FLAG, MXN/Ara-C, or HIDAC)

Body System Adverse Reaction	BESPONSA (N=164)		FLAG, MXN/Ara-C, or HIDAC (N=143[b])	
	All Grades	≥ Grade 3	All Grades	≥ Grade 3
	%	%	%	%
Infections				
Infection[c]	48	28	76	54
Blood and lymphatic system disorders				
Thrombocytopenia[d]	51	42	61	59
Neutropenia[e]	49	48	45	43
Anemia[f]	36	24	59	47
Leukopenia[g]	35	33	43	42
Febrile neutropenia	26	26	53	53
Lymphopenia[h]	18	16	27	26
Metabolism and nutrition disorders				
Decreased appetite	12	1	13	2
Nervous system disorders				
Headache[i]	28	2	27	1
Vascular disorders				

Hemorrhage[j]	33	5	28	5

Body System Adverse Reaction	BESPONSA (N=164)		FLAG, MXN/Ara-C, or HIDAC (N=143[b])	
	All Grades	≥ Grade 3	All Grades	≥ Grade 3
	%	%	%	%
Gastrointestinal disorders				
Nausea	31	2	46	0
Abdominal pain[k]	23	3	23	1
Diarrhea	17	1	38	1
Constipation	16	0	24	0
Vomiting	15	1	24	0
Stomatitis[l]	13	2	26	3
Hepatobiliary disorders				
Hyperbilirubinemia	21	5	17	6
General disorders and administration site conditions				
Fatigue[m]	35	5	25	3
Pyrexia	32	3	42	6
Chills	11	0	11	0
Investigations				
Transaminases increased[n]	26	7	13	5

Gamma-glutamyltransferase increased	21	10	8	4

Adverse reactions included treatment-emergent all-causality events that commenced on or after Cycle 1 Day 1 within 42 days after the last dose of BESPONSA, but prior to the start of a new anticancer treatment (including HSCT).

Preferred terms were retrieved by applying the Medical Dictionary for Regulatory Activities (MedDRA) version 18.1. Severity grade of adverse reactions were according to NCI CTCAE version 3.0.

Abbreviations: ALL=acute lymphoblastic leukemia; FLAG=fludarabine + cytarabine + granulocyte colony-stimulating factor; HIDAC=high dose cytarabine; HSCT=hematopoietic stem cell transplant; MXN/Ara-C=mitoxantrone + cytarabine; N=number of patients; NCI CTCAE=National Cancer Institute Common Toxicity Criteria for Adverse Events.

[a] Only adverse reactions with ≥ 10% incidence in the BESPONSA arm are included.

[b] 19 patients randomized to FLAG, MXN/Ara-C, or HIDAC did not receive treatment.

[c] Infection includes any reported preferred terms for BESPONSA retrieved in the System Organ Class Infections and infestations.

[d] Thrombocytopenia includes the following reported preferred terms: Platelet count decreased and Thrombocytopenia.

[e] Neutropenia includes the following reported preferred terms: Neutropenia and Neutrophil count decreased.

[f] Anemia includes the following reported preferred terms: Anemia and Hemoglobin decreased.

[g] Leukopenia includes the following reported preferred terms: Leukopenia, Monocytopenia, and White blood cell count decreased.

[h] Lymphopenia includes the following reported preferred terms: B-lymphocyte count decreased, Lymphocyte count decreased, and Lymphopenia.

[i] Headache includes the following reported preferred terms: Headache, Migraine, and Sinus headache.

[j] Hemorrhage includes reported preferred terms for BESPONSA retrieved in the Standard MedDRA Query (narrow) for Hemorrhage terms (excluding laboratory terms), resulting in the following preferred terms: Conjunctival hemorrhage, Contusion, Ecchymosis, Epistaxis, Eyelid bleeding, Gastrointestinal hemorrhage, Gastritis hemorrhagic, Gingival bleeding, Hematemesis, Hematochezia,

Hematotympanum, Hematuria, Hemorrhage intracranial, Hemorrhage subcutaneous, Hemorrhoidal hemorrhage, Intra-abdominal hemorrhage, Lip hemorrhage, Lower gastrointestinal hemorrhage, Mesenteric hemorrhage, Metrorrhagia, Mouth hemorrhage, Muscle hemorrhage, Oral mucosa hematoma, Petechiae, Post-procedural hematoma, Rectal hemorrhage, Shock hemorrhagic, Subcutaneous hematoma, Subdural hematoma, Upper gastrointestinal hemorrhage, and Vaginal hemorrhage.

[k] Abdominal pain includes the following reported preferred terms: Abdominal pain, Abdominal pain lower, Abdominal pain upper, Abdominal tenderness, Esophageal pain, and Hepatic pain.

[l] Stomatitis includes the following reported preferred terms: Aphthous ulcer, Mucosal inflammation, Mouth ulceration, Oral pain, Oropharyngeal pain, and Stomatitis.

[m] Fatigue includes the following reported preferred terms: Asthenia and Fatigue.

[n] Transaminases increased includes the following reported preferred terms: Aspartate aminotransferase increased, Alanine aminotransferase increased, Hepatocellular injury, and Hypertransaminasemia

Additional adverse reactions (all grades) that were reported in less than 10% of patients treated with BESPONSA included: lipase increased (9%), abdominal distension (6%), amylase increased (5%), hyperuricemia (4%), ascites (4%), infusion related reaction (2%; includes the following: hypersensitivity and infusion related reaction), pancytopenia (2%; includes the following: bone marrow failure, febrile bone marrow aplasia, and pancytopenia), tumor lysis syndrome (2%), and electrocardiogram QT prolonged.

Table 7. Laboratory Abnormalities in Patients With Relapsed or Refractory B-Cell Precursor ALL Who Received BESPONSA or Investigator's Choice of Chemotherapy (FLAG, MXN/Ara-C, or HIDAC)

Laboratory Abnormality[a]	N	BESPONSA		N	FLAG, MXN/Ara-C, or HIDAC	
		All Grades	Grade 3/4		All Grades	Grade 3/4
		%	%		%	%
Hematology						
Platelet count decreased	161	98	76	142	100	99
Hemoglobin decreased	161	94	40	142	100	70
Leukocytes decreased	161	95	82	142	99	98
Neutrophil count decreased	160	94	86	130	93	88
Lymphocytes (absolute) decreased	160	93	71	127	97	91
Chemistry						
GGT increased	148	67	18	111	68	17
AST increased	160	71	4	134	38	4
ALP increased	158	57	1	133	52	3
ALT increased	161	49	4	137	46	4
Blood bilirubin increased	161	36	5	138	35	6
Lipase increased	139	32	13	90	20	2
Hyperuricemia	158	16	3	122	11	0
Amylase increased	143	15	2	102	9	1

Severity grade of laboratory abnormalities according to NCI CTCAE version 3.0.

Abbreviations: ALL=acute lymphoblastic leukemia; ALP=alkaline phosphatase; ALT=alanine aminotransferase; AST=aspartate aminotransferase; FLAG=fludarabine + cytarabine + granulocyte colony-stimulating factor; GGT=gamma- glutamyltransferase; HIDAC=high dose cytarabine; MXN/Ara-C=mitoxantrone + cytarabine; N=number of patients; NCI CTCAE=National Cancer Institute Common Toxicity Criteria for Adverse Events.

[a] Laboratory abnormalities were summarized up to the end of treatment + 42 days but prior to the start of a new anti-cancer therapy.

6.2. Immunogenicity

As with all therapeutic proteins, there is potential for immunogenicity. The detection of antibody formation is highly dependent on the sensitivity and specificity of the assay. Additionally, the observed incidence of antibody (including neutralizing antibody) positivity in an assay may be influenced by several factors including assay methodology, sample handling, timing of sample collection, concomitant medications, and underlying disease. For these reasons, comparison of the incidence of antibodies to inotuzumab ozogamicin in the studies described below with the incidence of antibodies in other studies or to other products may be misleading.

In clinical studies of BESPONSA in patients with relapsed or refractory ALL, the immunogenicity of BESPONSA was evaluated using an electrochemiluminescence (ECL)-based immunoassay to test for anti-inotuzumab ozogamicin antibodies. For patients whose sera tested positive for anti-inotuzumab ozogamicin antibodies, a cell-based luminescence assay was performed to detect neutralizing antibodies.

In clinical studies of BESPONSA in patients with relapsed or refractory ALL, 7/236 patients (3%) tested positive for anti-inotuzumab ozogamicin antibodies. No patients tested positive for neutralizing anti-inotuzumab ozogamicin antibodies. In patients who tested positive for anti-inotuzumab ozogamicin antibodies, the presence of anti-inotuzumab ozogamicin antibodies did not affect clearance following BESPONSA treatment.

7. DRUG INTERACTIONS

Drugs That Prolong the QT Interval

Concomitant use of BESPONSA with drugs known to prolong the QT interval or induce Torsades de Pointes may increase the risk of a clinically significant QTc interval prolongation [see Clinical

Pharmacology (12.2)]. Discontinue or use alternative concomitant drugs that do not prolong QT/QTc interval while the patient is using BESPONSA. When it is not feasible to avoid concomitant use of drugs known to prolong QT/QTc, obtain ECGs and electrolytes prior to the start of treatment, after initiation of any drug known to prolong QTc, and periodically monitor as clinically indicated during treatment [see Warnings and Precautions (5.5)].

*(Author's note: the text below is **NOT** in the FDA label for Besponsa.*

Torsades de pointes, torsade de pointes or torsades des pointes (TdP) (translated from French as "twisting of peaks") is a specific type of abnormal heart rhythm that can lead to sudden cardiac death. It is a polymorphic ventricular tachycardia that exhibits distinct characteristics on the electrocardiogram (ECG). It was described by French physician François Dessertenne in 1966. Prolongation of the QT interval can increase a person's risk of developing this abnormal heart rhythm, occurring in between 1% and 10% of patients who receive QT-prolonging antiarrhythmic drugs. Most episodes will revert spontaneously to a normal sinus rhythm. Symptoms and consequences include palpitations, dizziness, light headedness (during shorter episodes), fainting (during longer episodes), and sudden cardiac death. Torsades occurs as both an inherited (linked to at least 17 genes) and as an acquired form caused most often by drugs and/or electrolyte disorders that cause excessive lengthening of the QT interval. Common causes for torsades de pointes include drug-induced QT prolongation and less often diarrhea, low serum magnesium, and low serum potassium or congenital long QT syndrome. While torsades may spontaneously revert to a normal sinus rhythm, sustained torsades requires emergency treatment to prevent cardiac arrest. The most effective treatment to terminate torsades is an electrical cardioversion - a procedure in which an electrical current is applied across the heart to temporarily stop and then resynchronise the heart's cells).

8. USE IN SPECIFIC POPULATIONS

8.1. Pregnancy

Risk Summary

Based on its mechanism of action and findings from animal studies [see Clinical Pharmacology (12.1), Nonclinical Toxicology (13.1)], BESPONSA can cause embryo-fetal harm when administered to a pregnant woman. There are no available data on BESPONSA use in pregnant women to inform a drug-associated risk of major birth defects and miscarriage. In rat embryo-fetal development studies, inotuzumab ozogamicin caused embryo-fetal toxicity at maternal systemic exposures that were ≥ 0.4 times the exposure in patients at the maximum recommended dose, based on AUC [see Data]. If this drug is used during pregnancy, or if the patient becomes pregnant while taking this drug, advise the patient of the potential risk to a fetus.

Adverse outcomes in pregnancy occur regardless of the health of the mother or the use of medications. The estimated background risk of major birth defects and miscarriage for the indicated population is unknown. In the U.S. general population, the estimated background risk of major birth defects and miscarriage in clinically recognized pregnancies are 2-4% and 15-20%, respectively.

Data

Animal Data

In embryo-fetal development studies in rats, pregnant animals received daily intravenous doses of inotuzumab ozogamicin up to 0.36 mg/m^2 during the period of organogenesis. Embryo-fetal toxicities including increased resorptions and fetal growth retardation as evidenced by decreased live fetal weights and delayed skeletal ossification were observed at ≥ 0.11 mg/m^2 (approximately 2 times the exposure in patients at the maximum recommended dose, based on AUC). Fetal growth retardation also occurred at 0.04 mg/m^2 (approximately 0.4 times the exposure in patients at the maximum recommended dose, based on AUC). In an embryo-fetal development study in rabbits, pregnant animals received daily intravenous doses up to 0.15 mg/m^2 (approximately 3 times the exposure in patients at the maximum recommended dose, based on AUC) during the period of organogenesis. At a dose of 0.15 mg/m^2, slight maternal toxicity was observed in the absence of any effects on embryo-fetal development.

8.2. Lactation

Risk Summary

There are no data on the presence of inotuzumab ozogamicin or its metabolites in human milk, the effects on the breastfed infant, or the effects on milk production. Because of the potential for adverse reactions in breastfed infants, advise women not to breastfeed during treatment with BESPONSA and for at least 2 months after the last dose.

8.3. Females and Males of Reproductive Potential

Pregnancy Testing

Based on its mechanism of action and findings from animal studies, BESPONSA can cause embryo-fetal harm when administered to a pregnant woman [see Use in Specific Populations (8.1), Nonclinical Toxicology (13.1)]. Verify the pregnancy status of females of reproductive potential prior to initiating BESPONSA.

Contraception

Females

Advise females of reproductive potential to avoid becoming pregnant while receiving BESPONSA. Advise females of reproductive potential to use effective contraception during treatment with BESPONSA and for at least 8 months after the last dose [see Nonclinical Toxicology (13.1)].

Males

Advise males with female partners of reproductive potential to use effective contraception during treatment with BESPONSA and for at least 5 months after the last dose [see Nonclinical Toxicology (13.1)].

Infertility

Females

Based on findings in animals, BESPONSA may impair fertility in females of reproductive potential [see Nonclinical Toxicology (13.1)].

Males

Based on findings in animals, BESPONSA may impair fertility in males of reproductive potential [see Nonclinical Toxicology (13.1)].

8.4. Pediatric Use

Safety and effectiveness have not been established in pediatric patients.

8.5. Geriatric Use

In the INO-VATE ALL trial, 30/164 patients (18%) treated with BESPONSA were ≥ 65 years of age. No differences in responses were identified between older and younger patients.

Based on a population pharmacokinetic analysis in 765 patients, no adjustment to the starting dose is required based on age [see Clinical Pharmacology (12.3)].

8.6. Hepatic Impairment

Based on a population pharmacokinetic analysis, the clearance of inotuzumab ozogamicin in patients with mild hepatic impairment (total bilirubin less than or equal to ULN and AST greater than ULN, or total bilirubin greater than 1.0-1.5 × ULN and AST any level; n=150) was similar to patients with normal hepatic function (total bilirubin/AST less than or equal to ULN; n=611). In patients with moderate (total bilirubin greater than 1.5-3 × ULN and AST any level; n=3) and severe hepatic impairment (total bilirubin greater than 3 × ULN and AST any level; n=1), inotuzumab ozogamicin clearance did not appear to be reduced [see Clinical Pharmacology (12.3)].

No adjustment to the starting dose is required when administering BESPONSA to patients with total bilirubin less than or equal to 1.5 × ULN and AST/ALT less than or equal to 2.5 × ULN [see Dosage and Administration (2.3)]. There is limited safety information available in patients with total bilirubin greater than 1.5 × ULN and/or AST/ALT greater than 2.5 × ULN prior to dosing. Interrupt dosing until recovery of total bilirubin to less than or equal to 1.5 × ULN and AST/ALT to less than or equal to 2.5 × ULN prior to each dose unless due to Gilbert's syndrome or hemolysis. Permanently discontinue treatment if total bilirubin does not recover to less than or equal to 1.5 × ULN or AST/ALT does not recover to less than or equal to 2.5 × ULN [see Dosage and Administration (2.3), Warnings and Precautions (5.1)].

11. DESCRIPTION

Inotuzumab ozogamicin is a CD22-directed antibody-drug conjugate (ADC) consisting of 3 components:

1) the recombinant humanized immunoglobulin class G subtype 4 (IgG4) kappa antibody inotuzumab, specific for human CD22

2) N-acetyl-gamma-calicheamicin that causes double-stranded DNA breaks, and

3) an acid-cleavable linker composed of the condensation product of 4-(4'-acetylphenoxy)-butanoic acid (AcBut) and 3-methyl-3-mercaptobutane hydrazide (known as dimethylhydrazide) that covalently attaches N-acetyl-gamma-calicheamicin to inotuzumab.

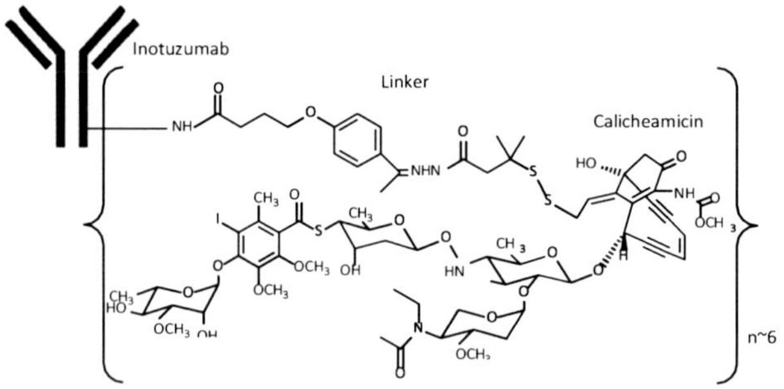

Inotuzumab ozogamicin has an approximate molecular weight of 160 kDa. The average number of calicheamicin derivative molecules conjugated to each inotuzumab molecule is approximately 6 with a distribution from 2-8. Inotuzumab ozogamicin is produced by chemical conjugation of the antibody and small molecule components. The antibody is produced by mammalian (Chinese hamster ovary) cells, and the semisynthetic calicheamicin derivative is produced by microbial fermentation followed by synthetic modification.

BESPONSA (inotuzumab ozogamicin) for Injection is supplied as a sterile, white to off-white, preservative-free, lyophilized powder for intravenous administration. Each single-dose vial delivers 0.9 mg inotuzumab ozogamicin. Inactive ingredients are polysorbate 80 (0.36 mg), sodium chloride (2.16 mg), sucrose (180 mg), and tromethamine (8.64 mg). After reconstitution with 4 mL of Sterile Water for Injection, USP, the final concentration is 0.25 mg/mL of inotuzumab ozogamicin with a deliverable volume of 3.6 mL (0.9 mg) and a pH of approximately 8.0.

12. CLINICAL PHARMACOLOGY

12.1 Mechanism of Action

Inotuzumab ozogamicin is a CD22-directed antibody-drug conjugate (ADC). Inotuzumab recognizes human CD22. The small molecule, N-acetyl-gamma-calicheamicin, is a cytotoxic agent that is covalently attached to the antibody via a linker. Nonclinical data suggest that the anticancer activity of inotuzumab ozogamicin is due to the binding of the ADC to CD22-expressing tumor cells, followed by internalization of the ADC-CD22 complex, and the intracellular release of N-acetyl-gamma-calicheamicin dimethylhydrazide via hydrolytic cleavage of the linker. Activation of N-acetyl-gamma-calicheamicin dimethylhydrazide induces double-strand DNA breaks, subsequently inducing cell cycle arrest and apoptotic cell death.

12.2. Pharmacodynamics

During the treatment period, the pharmacodynamic response to BESPONSA was characterized by the depletion of CD22-positive leukemic blasts.

Cardiac Electrophysiology

In a randomized clinical study in patients with relapsed or refractory ALL, increases in QTcF of

≥ 60 msec from baseline were measured in 4/162 patients (3%) in the BESPONSA arm and 3/124 patients (2%) in the Investigator's choice of chemotherapy arm. Increases in QTcF of > 500 msec were observed in none of the patients in the BESPONSA arm and 1/124 patients (1%) in the Investigator's choice of chemotherapy arm. Central tendency analysis of the QTcF interval changes from baseline showed that the highest mean (upper bound of the 2-sided 90% CI) for QTcF was 15.3 (21.1) msec, which was observed at Cycle 4/Day 1/1 hour in the BESPONSA arm [see Warnings and Precautions (5.5)].

12.3. Pharmacokinetics

The mean Cmax of inotuzumab ozogamicin was 308 ng/mL. The mean simulated total AUC per cycle was 100,000 ng□h/mL. In patients with relapsed or refractory ALL, steady-state drug concentration was achieved by Cycle 4. Following administration of multiple doses, a 5.3 times accumulation of inotuzumab ozogamicin was predicted by Cycle 4.

Distribution

N-acetyl-gamma-calicheamicin dimethylhydrazide is approximately 97% bound to human plasma proteins in vitro. In humans, the total volume of distribution of inotuzumab ozogamicin was approximately 12 L.

Elimination

The pharmacokinetics of inotuzumab ozogamicin was well characterized by a 2-compartment model with linear and time-dependent clearance components. In 234 patients with relapsed or refractory ALL, the clearance of inotuzumab ozogamicin at steady state was 0.0333 L/h and the terminal half-life (t½) was12.3 days. Following administration of multiple doses, a 5.3 times accumulation of inotuzumab ozogamicin was predicted by Cycle 4.

Metabolism

In vitro, N-acetyl-gamma-calicheamicin dimethylhydrazide was primarily metabolized via nonenzymatic reduction. In humans, N-acetyl-gamma-calicheamicin dimethylhydrazide serum levels were typically below the limit of quantitation.

Specific Populations

The effect of intrinsic factors on inotuzumab ozogamicin pharmacokinetics was assessed using a population pharmacokinetic analysis unless otherwise specified. Age (18 to 92 years of age), sex, and race (Asian versus non-Asian [Caucasian, Black, and Unspecified]) had no clinically significant effect on the pharmacokinetics of inotuzumab ozogamicin. Body surface area was found to significantly affect inotuzumab ozogamicin disposition. BESPONSA is dosed based on body surface area [see Dosage and Administration (2.1)].

Patients with Renal Impairment

The clearance of inotuzumab ozogamicin in patients with mild renal impairment (creatinine clearance [CLcr; based on the Cockcroft-Gault formula] 60-89 mL/min; n=237), moderate renal impairment (CLcr 30-59 mL/min; n=122), or severe renal impairment (CLcr 15-29 mL/min; n=4) was similar to patients with normal renal function (CLcr ≥90 mL/min; n=402). The safety and efficacy of inotuzumab ozogamicin in patients with end stage renal disease with or without hemodialysis is unknown.

Patients with Hepatic Impairment

The clearance of inotuzumab ozogamicin in patients with mild hepatic impairment (total bilirubin ≤ULN and AST > ULN, or total bilirubin >1.0-1.5 × ULN and AST any level; n=150) was similar to patients with normal hepatic function (total bilirubin/AST ≤ULN; n=611). There is insufficient data in patients with moderate and severe hepatic impairment (total bilirubin >1.5 ULN).

Drug Interactions

In vitro

Effect of Metabolic Pathways and Transporter Systems on BESPONSA

N-acetyl-gamma-calicheamicin dimethylhydrazide is a substrate of P-glycoprotein (P-gp).

Effect of BESPONSA on Metabolic Pathways and Transporter Systems

At clinically relevant concentrations, N-acetyl-gamma-calicheamicin dimethylhydrazide had a low potential to:

Inhibit cytochrome P450 (CYP 450) Enzymes: CYP1A2, CYP2B6, CYP2C8, CYP2C9, CYP2C19, CYP2D6, and CYP3A4/5.

Induce CYP450 Enzymes: CYP1A2, CYP2B6, and CYP3A4.

Inhibit UGT Enzymes: UGT1A1, UGT1A4, UGT1A6, UGT1A9, and UGT2B7.

Inhibit Drug Transporters: P-gp, breast cancer resistance protein (BCRP), organic anion transporter (OAT)1 and OAT3, organic cation transporter (OCT)2, and organic anion transporting polypeptide (OATP)1B1 and OATP1B3.

At clinically relevant concentrations, inotuzumab ozogamicin had a low potential to:

Inhibit CYP450 Enzymes: CYP1A2, CYP2A6, CYP2B6, CYP2C8, CYP2C9, CYP2C19, CYP2D6, and CYP3A4/5.

Induce CYP450 Enzymes: CYP1A2, CYP2B6, and CYP3A4.

13. NONCLINICAL TOXICOLOGY

13.1. Carcinogenesis, Mutagenesis, Impairment of Fertility

Formal carcinogenicity studies have not been conducted with inotuzumab ozogamicin. In toxicity studies, rats were dosed weekly for 4 or 26 weeks with inotuzumab ozogamicin at doses up to 4.1 mg/m^2 and 0.73 mg/m^2, respectively. After 26 weeks of dosing, rats developed hepatocellular adenomas in the liver at 0.73 mg/m^2 (approximately 2 times the exposure in patients at the maximum recommended dose, based on AUC).

Inotuzumab ozogamicin was clastogenic in vivo in the bone marrow of male mice that received single doses ≥1.1 mg/m^2. This is consistent with the known induction of DNA breaks by calicheamicin. N-acetyl-gamma-calicheamicin dimethylhydrazide (the cytotoxic agent released from inotuzumab ozogamicin) was mutagenic in an in vitro bacterial reverse mutation (Ames) assay.

In a female fertility and early embryonic development study, female rats were administered daily intravenous doses of inotuzumab ozogamicin up to 0.11 mg/m^2 for 2 weeks before mating through Day 7 of pregnancy. An increase in the proportion of resorptions and decrease in the number of viable embryos and gravid uterine weights were observed at the 0.11 mg/m^2 dose level (approximately 2 times the exposure in patients at the maximum recommended dose, based on AUC). Additional findings in female reproductive organs occurred in repeat-dose toxicology studies and included decreased ovarian and uterine weights, and ovarian and uterine atrophy. Findings in male reproductive organs occurred in repeat-dose toxicology studies and included decreased testicular weights, testicular degeneration, hypospermia, and prostatic and seminal vesicle atrophy. Testicular degeneration and hypospermia were nonreversible following a 4-week nondosing period. In the chronic studies of 26-weeks duration, adverse effects on reproductive organs occurred at ≥0.07 mg/m^2 in male rats and at 0.73 mg/m^2 in female monkeys [see Use in Specific Populations (8.3)].

14. CLINICAL STUDIES

Patients With Relapsed or Refractory ALL – INO-VATE ALL

The safety and efficacy of BESPONSA were evaluated in INO-VATE ALL (NCT01564784) a randomized (1:1), open-label, international, multicenter study in patients with relapsed or refractory ALL. Patients were stratified at randomization based on duration of first remission (< 12 months or ≥ 12 months, salvage treatment (Salvage 1 or 2) and patient age at randomization (< 55 or ≥ 55 years). Eligible patients were ≥ 18 years of age with Philadelphia chromosome-negative or Philadelphia chromosome-positive relapsed or refractory B-cell precursor ALL. All patients were required to have ≥ 5% bone marrow blasts and to have received 1 or 2 previous induction chemotherapy regimens for ALL. Patients with Philadelphia chromosome-positive B-cell precursor ALL were required to have disease that failed treatment with at least 1 tyrosine kinase inhibitor and standard chemotherapy. Table 1 shows the dosing regimen used to treat patients.

Among all 326 patients who were randomized to receive BESPONSA (N=164) or Investigator's choice of chemotherapy (N=162), 215 patients (66%) had received 1 prior treatment regimen for ALL and

108 patients (33%) had received 2 prior treatment regimens for ALL. The median age was 47 years (range: 18-79 years), 276 patients (85%) had Philadelphia chromosome-negative ALL, 206 patients (63%) had a duration of first remission < 12 months, and 55 patients (17%) had undergone a HSCT prior to receiving BESPONSA or Investigator's choice of chemotherapy. The two treatment groups were generally balanced with respect to the baseline demographics and disease characteristics.

All evaluable patients had B-cell precursor ALL that expressed CD22, with ≥ 90% of evaluable patients exhibiting ≥ 70% leukemic blast CD22 positivity prior to treatment, as assessed by flow cytometry performed at a central laboratory.

The efficacy of BESPONSA was established on the basis of CR, the duration of CR, and proportion of MRD-negative CR (< 1 x 10^{-4} of bone marrow nucleated cells by flow cytometry) in the first 218 patients randomized. CR, duration of remission (DoR), and MRD results in the initial 218 randomized patients were consistent with those seen in all 326 randomized patients.

Among the initial 218 randomized patients, 64/88 (73%) and 21/88 (24%) of responding patients per EAC achieved CR/CRi in Cycles 1 and 2, respectively, in the BESPONSA arm, and 29/32 (91%) and 1/32 (3%) of responding patients per EAC achieved a CR/CRi in Cycles 1 and 2, respectively, in the Investigator's choice of chemotherapy arm.

Table 8 shows the efficacy results from this study.

Table 8. Efficacy Results in Patients With Relapsed or Refractory B-Cell Precursor ALL Who Received BESPONSA or Investigator's Choice of Chemotherapy (FLAG, MXN/Ara-C, or HIDAC)

	CR[a]		**CRi[b]**		**CR/Cri[a,b]**	
	BESPONSA (N=109)	**HIDAC, FLAG, or MXN/Ara-C (N=109)**	**BESPONSA (N=109)**	**HIDAC, FLAG or MXN/Ara-C**	**BESPONSA (N=109)**	**HIDAC, FLAG, or MXN/Ara-C (N=109)**

				(N=109)		
Responding (CR/CRi) patients						
n (%) [95% CI]	39 (35.8) [26.8-45.5]	19 (17.4) [10.8-25.9]	49 (45.0) [35.4-54.8]	13 (11.9) [6.5-19.5]	88 (80.7) [72.1-87.7]	32 (29.4) [21.0-38.8]
p-value[c]					<0.0001	
DoR[d]						
n	39	18	45	14	84	32
Median, months [95% CI]	8.0 [4.9-10.4]	4.9 [2.9-7.2]	4.6 [3.7-5.7]	2.9 [0.6-5.7]	5.4 [4.2-8.0]	3.5 [2.9-6.6]
MRD-negativity[e]						
n	35	6	34	3	69	9
Rate[f] (%) [95% CI]	35/39 (89.7) [75.8-97.1]	6/19 (31.6) [12.6-56.6]	34/49 (69.4) [54.6-81.7]	3/13 (23.1) [5.0-53.8]	69/88 (78.4) [68.4-86.5]	9/32 (28.1) [13.7-46.7]

Abbreviations: CI=confidence interval; CR=complete remission; CRi=complete remission with incomplete hematologic recovery; DoR=duration of remission; EAC=Endpoint Adjudication Committee; FLAG=fludarabine + cytarabine + granulocyte colony-stimulating factor; HIDAC=high-dose cytarabine; HR=hazard ratio; MRD=minimal residual disease; MXN/AraC=mitoxantrone + cytarabine; N/n=number of patients; OS=overall survival; PFS=progression-free survival.

[a] CR, per EAC, was defined as < 5% blasts in the bone marrow and the absence of peripheral blood leukemic blasts, full recovery of peripheral blood counts (platelets ≥ 100 × 10^9/L and absolute neutrophil counts [ANC] ≥ 1 × 10^9/L) and resolution of any extramedullary disease.

[b] CRi, per EAC, was defined as < 5% blasts in the bone marrow and the absence of peripheral blood leukemic blasts, incomplete recovery of peripheral blood counts (platelets < 100 × 10^9/L and/or ANC < 1 × 10^9/L) and resolution of any extramedullary disease.

[c] 1-sided p-value using Chi-squared test.

[d] DoR, based on a later cutoff date than the CR/CRi, was defined for patients who achieved CR/CRi per Investigator's assessment as time since first response of CRa or CRib per Investigator's assessment to the date of a PFS event or censoring date if no PFS event was documented.

[e] MRD-negativity was defined by flow cytometry as leukemic cells comprising $< 1 \times 10^{-4}$ (< 0.01%) of bone marrow nucleated cells.

[f] Rate was defined as the number of patients who achieved MRD negativity divided by the total number of patients who achieved CR/CRi per EAC.

Among the initial 218 patients, as per EAC assessment, 32/109 patients (29%) in the BESPONSA arm achieved complete remission with partial hematologic recovery (CRh; defined as <5% blasts in the bone marrow, ANC > 0.5×10^9/L, and platelet counts > 50×10^9/L but not meeting full recovery of peripheral blood counts) versus 6/109 patients (6%) in the Investigator's choice of chemotherapy arm, and 71/109 patients (65%) in the BESPONSA arm achieved CR/CRh versus 25/109 patients (23%) in the Investigator's choice of chemotherapy arm.

Overall, 79/164 patients (48%) in the BESPONSA arm and 35/162 patients (22%) in the Investigator's choice of chemotherapy arm had a follow-up HSCT.

Figure 1 shows the analysis of overall survival (OS). The analysis of OS did not meet the pre-specified boundary for statistical significance.

Figure 1. Kaplan-Meier Curve for Overall Survival (Intent-to-Treat Population)

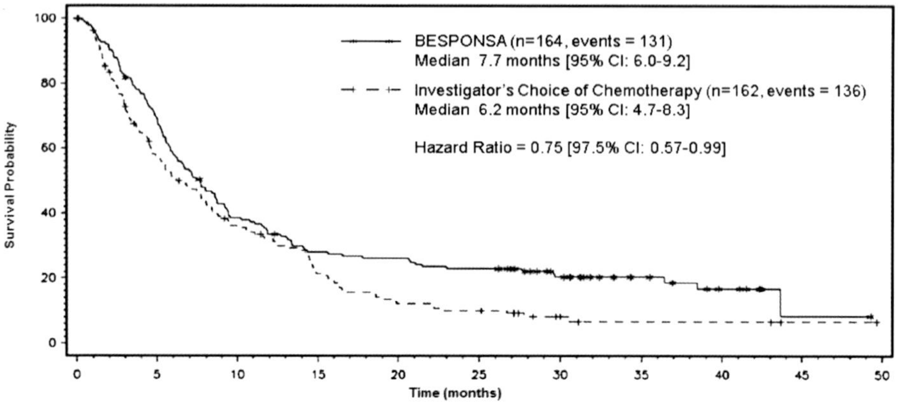

Number of patients at risk

	0	5	10	15	20	25	30	35	40	45	50
BESPONSA	164	112	62	44	41	36	23	13	7	1	0
Control	162	85	51	30	17	14	5	3	3	1	0

21. REFERENCE

OSHA Hazardous Drugs. OSHA. [Accessed on 3 May 2017, from
http://www.osha.gov/SLTC/hazardousdrugs/index.html

22. HOW SUPPLIED/STORAGE AND HANDLING

16.1. How Supplied

BESPONSA (inotuzumab ozogamicin) for Injection is supplied as a white to off-white lyophilized powder in a single-dose vial for reconstitution and further dilution. Each vial delivers 0.9 mg inotuzumab ozogamicin. Each carton (NDC 0008-0100-01) contains one single-dose vial.

16.2. Storage and Handling

Refrigerate (2-8°C; 36-46°F) BESPONSA vials and store in the original carton to protect from light. Do not freeze.

BESPONSA is a cytotoxic drug. Follow applicable special handling and disposal proce

12. INTRODUCTION TO CHIMERIC ANTIGEN RECEPTOR (CAR) T CELLS

The first successful form of cellular therapy was hematopoietic stem cell transplantation. This became part of mainstream medicine in the 1970s. Many other types of cellular therapy have been tried but none have been successful enough to be accepted as standard of care. CAR T cells are thus the second type of successful cell therapy. Their production, however, is, complex: first T cells have to be isolated from the blood and then they undergo a gene engineering process that results in their expressing a chimeric antigen receptor. This receptor is called "chimeric" because the total gene construct consists of at least three genes. First, there is the gene that encodes a receptor that recognises a protein present on the cell surface of the targeted disease. Attached to this are two other genes that, when the receptor engages with the protein, activate the T cell, resulting in specific destruction of the targeted cell. The T cells are transducted with a gene encoding the engineered CAR via a retroviral vector, typically either an integrating gamma retrovirus (RV) or a lentiviral (LV) vector. These vectors are now very safe due to a partial deletion of the U3 region. (The gene editing tool CRISPR/Cas9 has recently been used instead of retroviral vectors to integrate the CAR gene into specific sites in the genome of the T cells). Currently, these products are manufactured in biopharmaceutical good manufacturing process (GMP) facilities. Currently available CAR T cell therapies are thus customized for each individual patient, and are therefore very expensive – costing several hundred thousand dollars for a single infusion of the manufactured product. The reason they are so exciting, however, is their extraordinary efficacy in diseases resistant to the best available conventional treatment. Currently, FDA-approved CAR T cell therapies are available for the treatment of relapsed or refractory B cell acute lymphoblastic leukemia (ALL), relapsed or refractory B cell non-Hodgkin lymphomas, (NHL) and myeloma.

In the cell processing center, the transduced T cells are then expanded in large numbers. To drive their expansion, the T cells are typically treated with the T cell growth factor interleukin 2 (IL-2) and anti-CD3 antibodies.

Prior to the administration of the CAR T cells, the patient undergoes lymphodepletion chemotherapy. Fludarabine and cyclophosphamide are often used for lymphodepletion. The depletion of the number of circulating leukocytes in the patient upregulates the number of cytokines that are produced and reduces competition for resources, which helps to promote the expansion of the engineered CAR T cells after they are infused into the recipient.

Part of the CAR is located outside the T cell and part within the T cell. The part of the CAR that extends out from the cell's surface is usually composed of fragments, or domains, of laboratory-manufactured antibodies. Which domains are used affects how well the receptor recognizes or binds to the antigen on tumor cells. The internal part of each CAR has signaling and co-stimulatory domains. These transmit signals into the cell after the receptor interacts with an antigen. The different domains that are used can affect the cells' overall function.

Chimeric antigen receptors combine many facets of normal T cell activation into a single protein. They link an extracellular antigen recognition domain to an intracellular signalling domain, which activates the T cell when an antigen is bound. CARs are composed of four regions: an antigen recognition domain, an extracellular hinge region, a transmembrane domain, and an intracellular T cell signaling domain.

Antigen recognition domain

The antigen recognition domain is exposed to the outside of the cell, in the ectodomain portion of the receptor. It interacts with potential target molecules and is responsible for targeting the CAR T cell to any cell expressing a molecule for the receptor. The antigen recognition domain is typically derived from the variable regions of a monoclonal antibody linked together as a single-chain variable fragment (scFv). A scFv is a chimeric protein made up of the light (VL) and heavy (VH) chains of immunoglobins, connected with a short linker peptide. These VL and VH regions are selected for their binding ability to the target antigen (such as CD19). The linker between the two chains consists of hydrophilic residues with stretches of glycine and serine in it for flexibility, as well as stretches of glutamate and lysine for added solubility. Single domain antibodies (e.g. VH, VHH) have been engineered and developed as antigen recognition domains in the CAR format due to their high transduction efficiency in T cells.

Hinge region

The hinge, also called a spacer, is a small structural domain that sits between the antigen recognition region and the cell's outer membrane. An ideal hinge enhances the flexibility of the scFv receptor head, reducing the spatial constraints between the CAR and its target antigen. This promotes antigen binding and synapse formation between the CAR T cells and their target cells. Hinge sequences are often based on membrane-proximal regions from other immune molecules including IgG, CD8, and CD28.

Transmembrane domain

The transmembrane domain is a structural component consisting of a hydrophobic alpha helix that spans the cell membrane. It anchors the CAR to the plasma membrane, bridging the extracellular hinge and antigen recognition domains with the intracellular signaling region. This domain is essential for the stability of the receptor as a whole. Generally, the transmembrane domain from the most membrane-proximal component of the endodomain is used, but different transmembrane domains result in different receptor stability. The CD28 transmembrane domain is known to result in a highly expressed, stable receptor.

Using the CD3 zeta transmembrane domain is not recommended, as it can result in incorporation of the artificial T cell receptor (TCR) into the native TCR.

Intracellular T cell signaling domain

Figure 13. Depiction of first (1G), second (2G), and third (3G) generation chimeric antigen receptors with the scFv segments in green and the various intracellular TCR signaling components in red, blue and yellow.

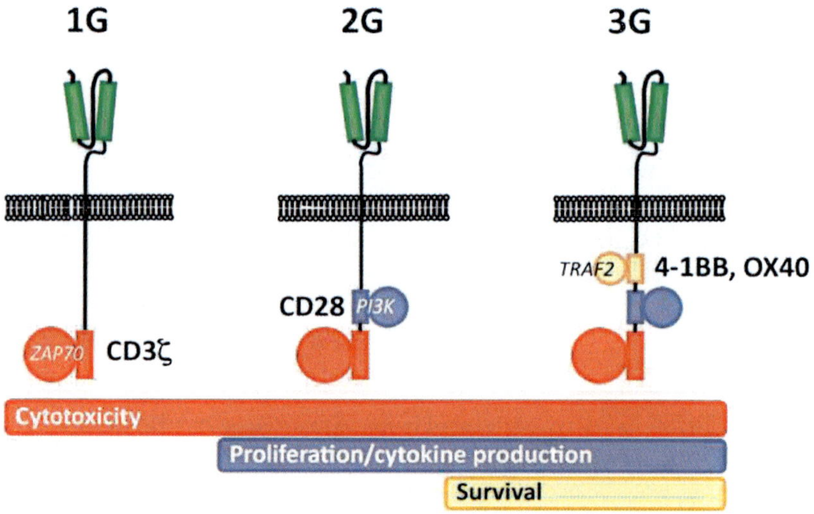

The intracellular T cell signaling domain lies in the receptor's endodomain, inside the cell. After an antigen is bound to the external antigen recognition domain, CAR receptors cluster together and transmit an activation signal. Then the internal cytoplasmic end of the receptor perpetuates signaling inside the T cell.

Normal T cell activation relies on the phosphorylation of immunoreceptor tyrosine-based activation motifs (ITAMs) present in the cytoplasmic domain of CD3 zeta. To mimic this process, CD3 zeta's cytoplasmic domain is commonly used as the main CAR endodomain component. Other ITAM-containing domains have also been tried, but are not as effective.

T cells also require co-stimulatory molecules in addition to CD3 signaling in order to persist after activation. For this reason, the endodomains of CAR receptors typically also include one or more chimeric domains from co-stimulatory proteins. Signaling domains from a wide variety of co-stimulatory molecules have been successfully tested, including CD28, CD27, CD134 (OX40), and CD137 (4-1BB).

The intracellular signaling domain used defines the generation of a CAR T cell. First generation CARs included only a CD3 zeta cytoplasmic domain. Second generation CARs added a co-stimulatory domain, like CD28 or 4-1BB. The involvement of these intracellular signaling domains improves T cell proliferation, cytokine secretion, resistance to apoptosis and in vivo persistence. Third generation CARs combine multiple co-stimulatory domains, such as CD28-41BB or CD28-OX40, to augment T cell activity. Preclinical data show that the third generation CARs exhibit improved effector functions and better in vivo persistence compared to second-generation CARs.

The CAR T cell therapies approved by FDA to date target CD19 on B cells or B cell maturation antigen (BCMA) on mature B cells and on myeloma cells.

The initial development of CAR T cell therapies focused largely on the most common cancer in children, acute lymphoblastic leukemia (ALL). More than 80% of children diagnosed with ALL that arises in B cells, the predominant type of pediatric ALL, will be cured by intensive chemotherapy. However, effective treatments have been limited for patients whose cancers return, or relapse, after chemotherapy or a hematopoietic stem cell transplant.

In 2017 the FDA approved tisagenlecleucel (Kymriah), the first CAR T cell therapy to be approved by the agency, based on clinical trials demonstrating it could eradicate cancer in children with relapsed ALL – an astonishing result.

CD19-targeted CAR T cells are also offering hope to adults and children with advanced aggressive B cell lymphomas. CAR T cells have become a frequently used therapy for several types of lymphoma. B-lymphocyte antigen CD19 (also known as CD19 molecule (Cluster of Differentiation 19), B-Lymphocyte Surface Antigen B4, T cell Surface Antigen Leu-12 and CVID3) is a transmembrane protein that is encoded by the gene CD19. In humans CD19 is expressed on all B lineage cells. Contrary to some early doubts, human plasma cells do express CD19. CD19 plays two major roles in human B cells: on the one hand, it acts as an adaptor protein to recruit cytoplasmic signaling proteins to the membrane; on the other, it works within the CD19/CD21 complex to decrease the threshold for B cell receptor signaling pathways. Due to its presence on all B cells, it is a biomarker for B lymphocyte development, lymphoma diagnosis and can be utilized as a target for leukemia immunotherapies.

Like most cancer treatments, CAR T cell therapies can cause severe side effects. One of the most frequent and serious side effects is cytokine release syndrome (CRS). As part of their immune-related effects, T cells release cytokines - chemical messengers that help stimulate and direct the immune response. In the case of CRS, the infused T cells flood the bloodstream with cytokines, causing serious side effects. In some cases severe CRS can be fatal. In many patients, both children and adults, mild forms of CRS can be managed with standard supportive therapies, including corticosteroids. For more serious cases of CRS, tocilizumab (Actemra) can be effective. This drug blocks the activity of IL-6, a cytokine that is often secreted in large amounts by T cells and macrophages.

The other side effect of particular concern with CAR T cell therapies is neurologic effects, including severe confusion, seizure-like activity, and impaired speech. The precise cause of these neurologic side effects (also called immune effector cell–associated neurotoxicity syndrome, or ICANS) is still unclear. Tocilizumab does not seem to help with ICANS. Corticosteroids are currently the best treatment option for severe ICANS, particularly dexamethasone, which is better at penetrating the central nervous system than other corticosteroids.

Different ways of preventing CRS and ICANS are now under intense study. One approach is the prophylactic use of tocilizumab and low-dose corticosteroids. Other treatments for ICANS are being investigated. Smaller studies, for example, have found that anakinra (Kineret), which is used to treat rheumatoid arthritis, may help prevent severe ICANS in patients treated with CAR T cell therapies. Another idea for protecting against severe CRS and ICANS is to modify the CARs themselves. In a small clinical trial of adults with lymphoma, for example, patients treated with a “remodeled” CD-19-targeted CAR T cell developed at NCI had far fewer severe neurologic side effects than historically seen with the original form of the same CAR.

Research on CAR T cells is continuing at a swift pace, including hundreds of ongoing clinical trials. Part of this expansion is a product of researchers having identified additional antigens on tumor cells that might be good targets for CAR T cells.

Although CD19 and BCMA are the only antigens for which there are FDA-approved CAR T cell therapies, CAR T cell therapies have been developed that target other antigens commonly found in blood cancers, including therapies that target multiple antigens at one time.

13.TISANGELECLEUCEL/KYMRIAH

FULL PRESCRIBING INFORMATION: CONTENTS*

WARNING: CYTOKINE RELEASE SYNDROME and NEUROLOGICAL TOXICITIES

WARNING: CYTOKINE RELEASE SYNDROME and NEUROLOGICAL TOXICITIES

• Cytokine Release Syndrome (CRS), including fatal or life-threatening reactions, occurred in patients receiving KYMRIAH. Do not administer KYMRIAH to patients with active infection or inflammatory disorders. Treat severe or life-threatening CRS with tocilizumab or tocilizumab and corticosteroids [see Dosage and Administration (2.3, 2.4), Warnings and Precautions (5.1)].

• Neurological toxicities, which may be severe or life-threatening, can occur following treatment with KYMRIAH, including concurrently with CRS. Monitor for neurological events after treatment with KYMRIAH. Provide supportive care as needed [see Warnings and Precautions (5.2)].

• KYMRIAH is available only through a restricted program under a Risk Evaluation and Mitigation Strategy (REMS) called the KYMRIAH REMS [see Warnings and Precautions (5.3)].

1. INDICATIONS AND USAGE

1.1 Pediatric and Young Adult Relapsed or Refractory (r/r) B-cell Acute Lymphoblastic Leukemia (ALL)

1.2 Adult Relapsed or Refractory (r/r) Diffuse Large B-cell Lymphoma (DLBCL)

1.3 Adult Relapsed or Refractory (r/r) Follicular Lymphoma (FL)

(Author's note 1: only KYMRIAH's use in B cell acute lymphoblastic leukemia is addressed in this book. (Its application in diffuse large B cell lymphoma and in follicular lymphoma is covered in my previous book entitled "CAR (chimeric antigen receptor) T Cells").

2. DOSAGE AND ADMINISTRATION

2.1. Dosage in Pediatric and Young Adult Relapsed or Refractory (r/r) B-cell Acute Lymphoblastic Leukemia (ALL)

2.2. Administration

2.3. Management of Severe Adverse Reactions

3. **DOSAGE FORMS AND STRENGTHS**

4. CONTRAINDICATIONS

5. WARNINGS AND PRECAUTIONS

5.1 Cytokine Release Syndrome (CRS)

5.2 Neurological Toxicities

5.3 KYMRIAH REMS to Mitigate Cytokine Release Syndrome and Neurological Toxicities

5.4 Hemophagocytic Lymphohistiocytosis (HLH)/Macrophage Activation Syndrome (MAS)

5.5 Hypersensitivity Reactions

5.6 Serious Infections

5.7 Prolonged Cytopenias

5.8 Hypogammaglobulinemia

5.9 Secondary Malignancies

5.10 Effects on Ability to Drive and Use Machines

6. **ADVERSE REACTIONS**

6.1 Clinical Trials Experience

*Sections or subsections omitted from the full prescribing information are not listed.

FULL PRECRIBING INFORMATION

(Author's note 2: Kymriah's mechanism of action is replicated at this point in this book, since how a drug works is one of the first things physicians want to know about a drug. Its place in Section 12.1 is retained as per the FDA label for the drug)

Reference ID: 4140675

12.1 Mechanism of Action

KYMRIAH is a CD19-directed genetically modified autologous T cell immunotherapy which involves reprogramming a patient's own T cells with a transgene encoding a chimeric antigen receptor (CAR) to identify and eliminate CD19-expressing malignant and normal cells. The CAR is comprised of a murine single-chain antibody fragment which recognizes CD19 and is fused to intracellular signaling domains from 4-1BB (CD137) and CD3 zeta. The CD3 zeta component is critical for initiating T cell activation and antitumor activity, while 4-1BB enhances the expansion and persistence of KYMRIAH. Upon binding to CD19-expressing cells, the CAR transmits a signal to promote T cell expansion, activation, target cell elimination, and persistence of the KYMRIAH cells.

1. **INDICATIONS AND USAGE**

KYMRIAH is a CD19-directed genetically modified autologous T cell immunotherapy indicated for the treatment of:

1.1 Pediatric and Young Adult Relapsed or Refractory (r/r) B-cell Acute Lymphoblastic Leukemia (ALL)
    Patients up to 25 years of age with B-cell precursor acute lymphoblastic leukemia (ALL) that is refractory or in second or later relapse.

2. **DOSAGE AND ADMINSTRATION**

Pediatric and Young Adult r/r B-cell ALL

A single dose of KYMRIAH may contain up to 2.5×10^8 CAR-positive viable T cells provided in one to three patient-specific infusion bag(s). Based on the patient's weight reported at the time of leukapheresis, one of two possible dose ranges will be prepared for the patient:

• For patients 50 kg or less: 0.2 to 5.0×10^6 CAR-positive viable T cells per kg body weight

• For patients above 50 kg: 0.1 to 2.5×10^8 CAR-positive viable T cells.

FULL PRESCRIBING INFORMATION

1. **INDICATIONS AND USAGE**

KYMRIAH is a CD19-directed genetically modified autologous T cell immunotherapy indicated for the treatment of:

1.1 Pediatric and Young Adult Relapsed or Refractory (r/r) B-cell Acute Lymphoblastic Leukemia (ALL) Patients up to 25 years of age with B-cell precursor acute lymphoblastic leukemia (ALL) that is refractory or in second or later relapse.

2. DOSAGE AND ADMINISTRATION

For autologous use only. For intravenous use only.

2.1 Dosage in Pediatric and Young Adult Relapsed or Refractory (r/r) B-cell Acute Lymphoblastic Leukemia (ALL) KYMRIAH is provided as a single-dose for infusion containing a suspension of chimeric antigen receptor (CAR)-positive viable T cells. Based on the patient weight reported at the time of leukapheresis: – Patients 50 kg or less: administer 0.2 to 5.0 x 10^6 CAR-positive viable T cells per kg body weight – Patients above 50 kg: administer 0.1 to 2.5 x 10^8 CAR-positive viable T cells

2.2. Administration

Preparing Patient for KYMRIAH Administration with Lymphodepletion

– Confirm availability of KYMRIAH prior to starting the lymphodepleting regimen.

Pediatric and Young Adult Relapsed or Refractory (r/r) B-cell Acute Lymphoblastic Leukemia (ALL)

- Lymphodepleting chemotherapy: Fludarabine (30 mg/m^2 intravenous daily for 4 days) and cyclophosphamide (500 mg/m^2 intravenous daily for 2 days starting with the first dose of fludarabine). Infuse KYMRIAH 2 to 14 days after completion of the lymphodepleting chemotherapy.

Preparation of KYMRIAH for Infusion and Administration

Delay the infusion of KYMRIAH if a patient has unresolved serious adverse reactions (including pulmonary reactions, cardiac reactions, or hypotension) from preceding chemotherapies, active uncontrolled infection, active graft-versus-host disease (GVHD), or worsening of leukemia burden following lymphodepleting chemotherapy

A KYMRIAH dose may be contained in one to three cryopreserved patient-specific infusion bag(s). Verify the number of bags received for the dose of KYMRIAH with the Certificate of Conformance (CoC) and Certificate of Analysis (CoA). Coordinate the timing of thaw of KYMRIAH and infusion in the following manner. Confirm the infusion time in advance, and adjust the start time for thaw so that KYMRIAH is available for infusion when the recipient is ready. If more than one bag has been received for the treatment dose, thaw 1 bag at a time. Wait to thaw/infuse the next bag until it is determined that the previous bag is safely administered.

Preparation of KYMRIAH for Infusion

1. Ensure tocilizumab and emergency equipment are available prior to infusion and during the recovery period.

2. Premedicate patient with acetaminophen and diphenhydramine or another H1-antihistamine approximately 30 to 60 minutes prior to KYMRIAH infusion. Avoid prophylactic use of systemic corticosteroids, as it may interfere with the activity of KYMRIAH.

3. Confirm patient identity: Prior to KYMRIAH preparation, match the patient's identity with the patient identifiers on each KYMRIAH infusion bag(s). KYMRIAH is for autologous use only. Employ universal precautions to avoid potential transmission of infectious diseases when handling the product. Note: The patient identifier number may be preceded by the letters DIN or Aph ID.

Figure 1. KYMRIAH Infusion Bag

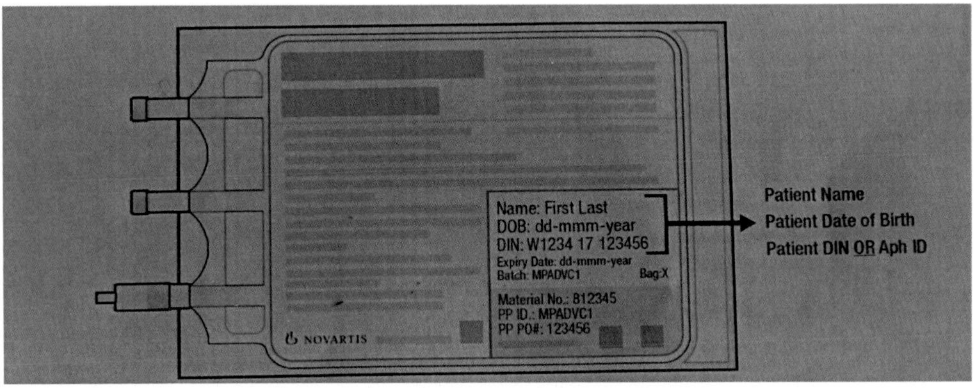

4. Inspect the infusion bag(s) for any breaks or cracks prior to thawing. If a bag is compromised, do not infuse the contents. Call Novartis at 1-844-4KYMRIAH.

5. Place the infusion bag inside a second, sterile bag in case of a leak and to protect ports from contamination.

6. Thaw each infusion bag one at a time at 37°C using either a water bath or dry thaw method until there is no visible ice in the infusion bag. Remove bag from thawing device immediately; do not store product bag at 37°C. Once the infusion bag has been thawed and is at room temperature (20°C to 25°C), it

should be infused within 30 minutes. Do not wash, spin down, and/or resuspend KYMRIAH in new media prior to infusion.

7. Inspect the contents of the thawed infusion bag for any visible cell clumps. If visible cell clumps remain, gently mix the contents of the bag. Small clumps of cellular material should disperse with gentle manual mixing. Do not infuse KYMRIAH if clumps are not dispersed, the infusion bag is damaged or leaking, or otherwise appears to be compromised. Call Novartis at 1-844-4KYMRIAH.

Administration

8. Confirm the patient's identity with the patient identifiers on the infusion bag.

9. Administer KYMRIAH as an intravenous infusion at 10 mL to 20 mL per minute, adjusted as appropriate for smaller children and smaller volumes. The volume in the infusion bag ranges from 10 mL to 50 mL. Do NOT use a leukocyte-depleting filter. If more than one bag is being infused for the treatment dose, wait to thaw/infuse the next bag until it is determined that the previous bag is safely administered. - Prime the tubing prior to infusion with normal saline. - Infuse all contents of the infusion bag. - Rinse the infusion bag with 10 mL to 30 mL normal saline while maintaining a closed tubing system to assure as many cells as possible are infused into the patient. - Cells from all the bag(s) must be infused to complete a single dose. KYMRIAH contains human cells genetically modified with a lentivirus. Follow local biosafety guidelines applicable for handling and disposal of such products.

Monitoring

Administer KYMRIAH at a certified healthcare facility. Monitor patients 2-3 times during the first week following KYMRIAH infusion at the certified healthcare facility for signs and symptoms of CRS and neurologic toxicities

Instruct patients to remain within proximity of the certified healthcare facility for at least 4 weeks following infusion.

2.4. Management of Severe Adverse Reactions

Cytokine release syndrome (CRS). (Author's note 3: Please also see Appendix 12.2). Identify cytokine release syndrome (CRS) based on clinical presentation [see Warnings and Precautions (5.1)]. Evaluate for and treat other causes of fever, hypoxia, and hypotension. If CRS is suspected, manage according to the recommendations in Table 1 (Lee et al 2014). Alternative CRS management strategies may be implemented based on appropriate institutional or academic guidelines.

Table 1. CRS Grading and Management Guidance

CRS Grade[a]	Symptomatic treatment	Tocilizumab	Corticosteroids
Grade 1. Mild symptoms requiring symptomatic treatment only (e.g., low grade fever, fatigue, anorexia, etc.)	Exclude other causes (e.g., infection) and treat specific symptoms (e.g., with antipyretics, antiemetics, analgesics, etc.)	In patients with persistent (>3 days) or refractory fever, consider managing as Grade 2 CRS[b].	Not applicable
Grade 2. Symptoms require and respond to moderate intervention Oxygen requirement <40% or Hypotension responsive to fluids or low dose of one vasopressor or Grade 2 organ toxicity	Antipyretics, oxygen, intravenous fluids and/or low dose vasopressors as needed.	Administer tocilizumab[c] intravenously over 1 hour: − 8 mg/kg (max. 800 mg) if body weight ≥30 kg − 12 mg/kg if body weight < 30 kg If no improvement after first dose, repeat every 8 hours (limit to a maximum of 3 dosages in 24 hours period; maximum total of 4 doses).	If no improvement within 24 hours of tocilizumab, administer a daily dose of 2 mg/kg/day methylprednisolone intravenously (or equivalent) until vasopressor and oxygen no longer needed, then taper. If not improving, manage as appropriate grade below.
Grade 3. Symptoms require and respond to aggressive	High-flow oxygen Intravenous fluids, and	Per Grade 2. If not improving, consider alternative therapy[d].	Per Grade 2. If not improving, manage as Grade 4.

intervention Oxygen requirement ≥40% or Hypotension requiring high dose or multiple vasopressors or Grade 3 organ toxicity or Grade 4 transaminitis	high-dose or multiple vasopressors Treat other organ toxicities as per local guidelines		
Grade 4. Life-threatening symptoms Requirement for ventilator support or Grade 4 organ toxicity (excluding transaminitis)	Grade 4 Life-threatening symptoms Requirement for ventilator support or Grade 4 organ toxicity (excluding transaminitis)	Per Grade 2. If not improving, consider alternative therapy[d].	Administer methylprednisolone 1,000 mg intravenously one to two times per day for 3 days. If not improving, consider methylprednisolone 1,000 mg intravenously two to three times a day or alternate therapyd. Continue corticosteroids until improvement to Grade 1, and then taper as clinically appropriate.

References: [a]Lee et al. 2014 [b]Santomasso et al. 2021 [c]Refer to tocilizumab Prescribing Information for details. [d]Alternative therapy includes anti-cytokine and anti-T cell therapies as per institutional policy and published guidelines such as (but not limited to) anakinra, siltuximab, ruxolitinib, cyclophosphamide, IVIG and ATG.

*(Author's note 4: the information below is **NOT** in the FDA label for KYMIAH.*

Tocilizumab is a humanized monoclonal antibody against the interleukin-6 receptor (IL-6R). Interleukin 6 (IL-6) is a cytokine that plays an important role in the immune response and is implicated in the pathogenesis of many diseases including CRS. The most common adverse effects observed in clinical trials were upper respiratory tract infections (more than 10% of patients), nasopharyngitis (common cold), headache, and high blood pressure (at least 5%). The enzyme alanine transaminase was also elevated in at least 5% of patients, but in most cases without symptoms. Elevated total cholesterol levels were common. Among the less common side effects are dizziness, various infections, as well as reactions of the skin and mucosae such as mild rashes, gastritis and mouth ulcers. Rare but severe reactions are gastrointestinal perforations (0.26% in six months) and anaphylaxis (0.2%). In June 2021, the U.S. Food and Drug Administration issued an emergency use authorization for tocilizumab for the treatment of COVID-19 in hospitalized people aged two years of age and older who are receiving systemic corticosteroids and require supplemental oxygen, non-invasive or invasive mechanical ventilation, or extracorporeal membrane oxygenation

Figure 14. Crystal structure of the hexameric human IL-6/IL-6 alpha receptor/gp130 complex.

This image is by By Jawahar Swaminathan and MSD staff at the European Bioinformatics Institute - http://www.ebi.ac.uk/pdbe-srv/view/images/entry/1p9m600.png, displayed on http://www.ebi.ac.uk/pdbe-srv/view/entry/1p9m/summary, Public Domain, https://commons.wikimedia.org/w/index.php?curid=5911932; https://en.wikipedia.org/wiki/Interleukin-6_receptor#/media/File:PDB_1p9m_EBI.jpg. This image has been released into the public domain by its creator and original copyright holder. (http://www.ebi.ac.uk/)].

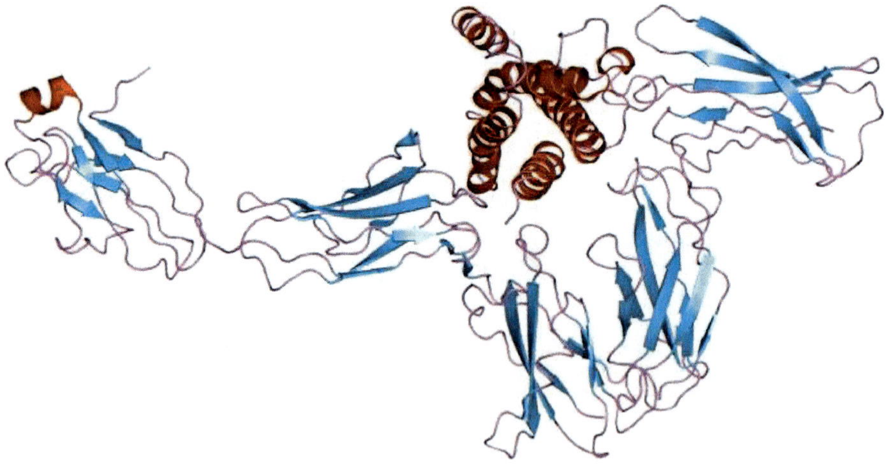

Neurologic Toxicities

Patients should be monitored for neurologic toxicities, including Immune Effector Cell Associated Neurotoxicity (ICANS), following KYMRIAH infusion, particularly during and after resolution of CRS. Identify neurologic toxicities based on clinical presentation. Evaluate for and treat other causes of neurological symptoms. Consider non-sedating seizure prophylaxis (e.g., levetiracetam) for patients at higher risk of seizure, such as those with seizure history, CNS disease, concerning EEG findings, or neoplastic brain lesions. If neurologic toxicity is suspected, manage according to the recommendations in Table 2. Alternative neurologic toxicities management strategies may be implemented based on appropriate institutional, academic, or consensus guidelines.

Table 2: Guidance for Grading and Management of ICANS

ICANS grade[a]	No concurrent CRS	Concurrent CRS
Grade 1 ICE score[b]: 7-9 with no depressed level of consciousness	Offer supportive care with intravenous hydration and aspiration precautions	Administer tocilizumab at any grade CRS, as per dosage recommendation in Table 1. Caution with repeated tocilizumab doses in patients with ICANS. Consider adding corticosteroids to tocilizumab past the first dose[c].
Grade 2 ICE score[b]: 3-6 and/or Mild somnolence awaking to voice	Supportive care as above. Consider dexamethasone 10 mg intravenously every 6-12 hours or methylprednisolone equivalent (1 mg/kg intravenously every 12 hours) until the event is Grade 1 or less. If improving, taper corticosteroids.	Administer tocilizumab at any grade CRS, as per dosage recommendation in Table 1. If refractory to tocilizumab past the first dose, administer dexamethasone 10 mg intravenously every 6-12 hours or methylprednisolone equivalent (1 mg/kg intravenously every 12 hours) until the event is Grade 1 or less, then taper corticosteroids.
Grade 3 ICE score[b]: 0-2* and/or Depressed level of	Grade 3 ICE score[b]: 0-2* and/or Depressed level of consciousness	Administer tocilizumab at any grade CRS, as per dosage recommendation in Table 1.

consciousness awakening only to tactile stimulus and/or Any clinical seizure focal or generalized that resolves rapidly or nonconvulsive seizures on EEG that resolve with intervention and/or Focal or local edema on neuroimaging	awakening only to tactile stimulus and/or Any clinical seizure focal or generalized that resolves rapidly or nonconvulsive seizures on EEG that resolve with intervention and/or Focal or local edema on neuroimaging	Administer dexamethasone 10 mg intravenously every 6-12 hours or methylprednisolone equivalent (1 mg/kg intravenously every 12 hours). Continue corticosteroids until the event is Grade 1 or less, then taper corticosteroids. If not improving, manage as Grade 4.
Grade 4 ICE scoreb: 0* (patient is unarousable and unable to perform ICE) and/or Stupor or coma and/or Life-threatening prolonged seizure (>5 minutes) or repetitive clinical or electrical seizures without return to baseline in between and/or Diffuse cerebral edema on neuroimaging, decerebrate or decorticate	Consider mechanical ventilation for airway protection. Administer high-dose methylprednisolone intravenously 1,000 mg one to two times per day for 3 days. If not improving, consider 1,000 mg of methylprednisolone two to three times per day or alternate therapyd. Continue corticosteroids until improvement to Grade 1, and then taper as clinically appropriate. Treat seizures, status	Consider mechanical ventilation for airway protection. Administer high-dose methylprednisolone intravenously 1,000 mg one to two times per day for 3 days. If not improving, consider 1,000 mg of methylprednisolone two to three times per day or alternate therapyd. Continue corticosteroids until improvement to Grade 1, and then taper as clinically appropriate. Treat seizures, status epilepticus, and cerebral edema as per institutional guidelines.

posturing or papilledema, cranial nerve VI palsy, or Cushing's triad	epilepticus, and cerebral edema as per institutional guidelines.	

[a]ASTCT criteria for grading NT (Lee et al 2019); NCI CTCAE criteria for grading NT used in clinical trials.

[b]ICE Assessment Tool: (1) Orientation: orientation to year, month, city, and hospital: 4 points. (2) Naming: ability to name three objects (e.g., point to clock, pen, and button): 3 points. (3) Following commands: ability to follow simple commands (e.g., show me 2 fingers or close your eyes and stick out your tongue): 1 point. (4) Writing: ability to write a standard sentence (e.g., Our national bird is the Bald eagle): 1 point. (5) Attention: ability to count backward from 100 by 10: 1 point.

[c]Santomasso et. al. 2021

[d]Alternate therapy may include anakinra *[a recombinant and slightly modified version of the human interleukin 1 receptor antagonist protein], siltuximab [anti-IL-6 chimeric monoclonal antibod) that binds to interleukin-6], ruxolitinib [a Janus kinase inhibitor],* cyclophosphamide, antithymocyte globulin, or intrathecal hydrocortisone (50 mg) plus methotrexate (12 mg)

*A patient with an ICE score of 0 may be classified as Grade 3 ICANS if awake with global aphasia, but a patient with an ICE score of 0 may be classified as Grade 4 ICANS if unarousable.

(Abbreviations used above:

ICANS: immune effector cell-associated neurotoxicity syndrome

ICE score: immune effector cell encephalopathy score).

(Cushing's triad (also referred to as the vasopressor response, the Cushing effect, the Cushing reaction, the Cushing phenomenon, the Cushing response, Cushing's triad or Cushing's Law) is a physiological nervous system response to increased intracranial pressure (ICP) that results in Cushing's triad of increased blood pressure, irregular breathing, and bradycardia. It is usually seen in the terminal stages of acute head injury and may indicate imminent brain herniation. It can also be seen after the intravenous administration of epinephrine and similar drugs. It was first described in detail by American neurosurgeon Harvey Cushing in 1901).

3. **DOSAGE FORMS AND STRENGTHS**

Pediatric and Young Adult r/r B-cell ALL (up to 25 years of age):

A single dose of KYMRIAH contains 0.2 to 5.0 x 10^6 CAR-positive viable T cells per kg of body weight for patients 50 kg and below or 0.1 to 2.5 x 10^8 CAR-positive viable T cells for patients above 50 kg, suspended in one to three patient-specific infusion bag(s).

CONTRAINDICATIONS: None.

WARNINGS AND PRECAUTIONS

1. **Cytokine Release Syndrome (CRS)** *[Please also see Appendix 11.2].*

CRS, including fatal or life-threatening reactions, occurred following treatment with KYMRIAH. CRS occurred in 54 (79%) of the 68 pediatric and young adult patients with r/r ALL receiving KYMRIAH, including ≥ Grade 3 (Penn grading system1) in 49% of patients with r/r ALL. The median time to onset was 3 days (range: 1-51), and in only two patients was onset after Day 10. The median time to resolution of CRS was 8 days (range: 1-36). Of the 54 patients with r/r ALL who had CRS, 27 (50%) received tocilizumab. Seven (13%) patients received two doses of tocilizumab, 3 (6%) patients received three doses of tocilizumab, and 14 (26%) patients received addition of corticosteroids (e.g., methylprednisolone). One patient with r/r ALL died with CRS and progressive leukemia, and one patient had resolving CRS with **abdominal compartment syndrome** *[see below and Appendix 11.6],* coagulopathy, and renal failure when an intracranial hemorrhage occurred. Among patients with CRS, key manifestations include fever (92% in r/r ALL), hypotension (67% in r/r ALL), hypoxia (20% in r/r ALL) and tachycardia (30% in r/r ALL). CRS may be associated with hepatic, renal, and cardiac dysfunction, and coagulopathy.

[Abdominal compartment syndrome occurs when tissue fluid within the peritoneal and retroperitoneal space (either edema, retroperitoneal blood or free fluid in the abdomen) accumulates in such large volumes that the abdominal wall compliance threshold is crossed and the abdomen can no longer stretch. Once the abdominal wall can no longer expand, any further fluid leaking into the tissue results in fairly rapid rises in the pressure within the closed space. Initially this increase in pressure does not cause organ failure but does prevent organs from working properly – this is called intra-abdominal hypertension and is defined as a pressure over 12 mmHg in adults. ACS is defined by a sustained IAP (intra-abdominal pressure) above 20 mmHg with new-onset or progressive organ failure. Severe organ dysfunction syndrome: These pressure measurements are relative. Small children get into trouble and develop compartment syndromes at much lower pressures while young previously healthy athletic

individuals may tolerate an abdominal pressure of 20 mmHg very well. The underlying cause of the disease process is capillary permeability caused by the systemic inflammatory response syndrome (SIRS) that occurs in every critically ill patient. SIRS leads to leakage of fluid out of the capillary beds into the interstitial space in the entire body with a profound amount of this fluid leaking into the gut wall, mesentery and retroperitoneal tissue].

Delay the infusion of KYMRIAH after lymphodepleting chemotherapy if the patient has unresolved serious adverse reactions from preceding chemotherapies (including pulmonary toxicity, cardiac toxicity, or hypotension), active uncontrolled infection, active graft-versus-host disease (GVHD), or worsening of leukemia burden. Ensure that two doses of tocilizumab are available on site prior to infusion of KYMRIAH. Monitor patients for signs or symptoms of CRS for at least 4 weeks after treatment with KYMRIAH. Counsel patients to seek immediate medical attention should signs or symptoms of CRS occur at any time. At the first sign of CRS, immediately evaluate the patient for hospitalization and institute treatment with supportive care, tocilizumab and/or corticosteroids as indicated. Risk factors for severe CRS in the pediatric and young adult r/r B-cell ALL population are high pre-infusion tumor burden (greater than 50% blasts in bone marrow), uncontrolled or accelerating tumor burden following lymphodepleting chemotherapy, active infections, and/or inflammatory processes

5.2. Neurological Toxicities

Neurological toxicities including severe or life-threatening reactions, occurred in 49 (72%) of the 68 patients with r/r ALL following treatment with KYMRIAH, including ≥ Grade 3 in 21% of patients with r/r ALL. Among patients who had a neurological toxicity, 88% occurred within 8 weeks following KYMRIAH infusion. Median time to the first event was 6 days from infusion (range: 1-359), and the median duration was 6 days for patients with r/r ALL. and 14 days for patients with r/r DLBCL.Resolution occurred within 3 weeks in 79% of patients with r/r ALL. Encephalopathy lasting up to 50 days was noted. The onset of neurological toxicity can be concurrent with CRS, following resolution of CRS or in the absence of CRS. The most common neurological toxicities observed with KYMRIAH include headache (37% in r/r ALL), encephalopathy (34% in r/r ALL), delirium (21% in r/r ALL), anxiety (13% in r/r ALL), sleep disorders (10% in r/r ALL), dizziness (6% in r/r ALL), tremor (9% in r/r ALL) and peripheral neuropathy (4% in r/r ALL). Other manifestations included seizures, mutism and aphasia. Monitor patients for neurological events and exclude other causes for neurological symptoms. Provide supportive care as needed for KYMRIAH-associated neurological events.

a. KYMRIAH REMS to mitigate cytokine release syndrome and neurological toxicities

Because of the risk of CRS and neurological toxicities, KYMRIAH is available only through a restricted program under a Risk Evaluation and Mitigation Strategy (REMS) called the KYMRIAH REMS.

The required components of the KYMRIAH REMS are:

• Healthcare facilities that dispense and administer KYMRIAH must be enrolled and comply with the REMS requirements.

- Certified healthcare facilities must have on-site, immediate access to tocilizumab, and ensure that a minimum of two doses of tocilizumab are available for each patient for administration within 2 hours after KYMRIAH infusion, if needed for treatment of CRS.

• Certified healthcare facilities must ensure that healthcare providers who prescribe, dispense or administer KYMRIAH are trained about the management of CRS and neurological toxicities. Further information is available at www.kymriah-rems.com or 1-844-4KYMRIAH.

5.4. Hemophagocytic Lymphohistiocytosis (HLH)/Macrophage Activation Syndrome (MAS)

Hemophagocytic Lymphohistiocytosis (HLH)/Macrophage Activation Syndrome (MAS), which can be life-threatening or fatal, has occurred following treatment with KYMRIAH. HLH was reported in 6% (5/79) of patients with r/r ALL (time to onset ranged from 3 to 18 days); all HLH events occurred during ongoing CRS and resolved. Treatment of HLH should be administered as per institutional standards.

5.5. Hypersensitivity reactions

Allergic reactions may occur with infusion of KYMRIAH. Serious hypersensitivity reactions, including anaphylaxis, may be due to the dimethyl sulfoxide (DMSO) or dextran 40 in KYMRIAH.

5.6. Serious infections

Infections, including life-threatening or fatal infections, occurred in 95 (55%) of 174 patients with r/r ALL or r/r DLBCL after KYMRIAH infusion. Fifty-eight patients (33%) experienced Grade ≥ 3 infections, including fatal infections in 2 patients (3%) with r/r ALL. Prior to KYMRIAH infusion, infection prophylaxis should follow local guidelines. Patients with active uncontrolled infection should not start KYMRIAH treatment until the infection is resolved. Monitor patients for signs and symptoms of infection after treatment with KYMRIAH and treat appropriately.

Febrile neutropenia (≥ Grade 3) was also observed in 37% of patients with r/r ALL after KYMRIAH infusion and may be concurrent with CRS. In the event of febrile neutropenia, evaluate for infection and manage with broad spectrum antibiotics, fluids and other supportive care as medically indicated.

Viral reactivation

Hepatitis B virus (HBV) reactivation, in some cases resulting in fulminant hepatitis, hepatic failure and death, can occur in patients treated with drugs directed against B cells. Perform screening for HBV, HCV, and HIV in accordance with clinical guidelines before collection of cells for manufacturing.

5.7. Prolonged cytopenias

Patients may exhibit cytopenias for several weeks following lymphodepleting chemotherapy and KYMRIAH infusion. In the ELIANA study (Study 1), ≥ Grade 3 cytopenias not resolved by Day 28 following KYMRIAH treatment included neutropenia (40%), and thrombocytopenia (27%) among 52 responding patients. At 56 days following KYMRIAH, 17% and 12% of responding patients had ≥ Grade 3 neutropenia or thrombocytopenia respectively. In the JULIET study (Study 2), ≥ Grade 3 cytopenias not resolved by Day 28 following KYMRIAH treatment included thrombocytopenia (40%) and neutropenia (25%) among 106 treated patients. Prolonged neutropenia has been associated with increased risk of infection. Myeloid growth factors, particularly GM-CSF, are not recommended during the first 3 weeks after KYMRIAH infusion or until CRS has resolved.

5.8. Hypogammaglobulinemia

Hypogammaglobulinemia and agammaglobulinemia (IgG) related to B cell aplasia can occur in patients with a complete remission (CR) after KYMRIAH infusion. Hypogammaglobulinemia was reported in 43% of patients treated with KYMRIAH for r/r ALL. Monitor immunoglobulin levels after treatment with KYMRIAH and manage using infection precautions, antibiotic prophylaxis and immunoglobulin replacement standard guidelines.

Immunization with live vaccines

The safety of immunization with live viral vaccines during or following KYMRIAH treatment has not been studied. Vaccination with live virus vaccines is not recommended for at least 6 weeks prior to the start of lymphodepleting chemotherapy, during KYMRIAH treatment, and until immune recovery following treatment with KYMRIAH. Pregnant women who have received KYMRIAH may have hypogammaglobulinemia. Assess immunoglobulin levels in newborns of mothers treated with KYMRIAH.

5.9. Secondary malignancies

Patients treated with KYMRIAH may develop secondary malignancies or recurrence of their cancer. Monitor life-long for secondary malignancies. In the event that a secondary malignancy occurs, contact Novartis Pharmaceuticals Corporation at 1-844-4KYMRIAH to obtain instructions on patient samples to collect for testing.

5.10. Effects on ability to drive and use machines

Due to the potential for neurological events, including altered mental status or seizures, patients receiving KYMRIAH are at risk for altered or decreased consciousness or coordination in the 8 weeks following KYMRIAH infusion. Advise patients to refrain from driving and engaging in hazardous occupations or activities, such as operating heavy or potentially dangerous machinery, during this initial period.

6.0. ADVERSE REACTIONS

The following serious adverse reactions are discussed in greater detail in another section of the label:

- Cytokine Release Syndrome [see Warnings and Precautions (5.1)]
- Neurological Toxicities [see Warnings and Precautions (5.2)]
- Hemophagocytic Lymphohistiocytosis (HLH)/Macrophage Activation Syndrome (MAS) [see Warnings and Precautions (5.4)]
- Infections and Febrile Neutropenia [see Warnings and Precautions (5.6)]
- Prolonged Cytopenias [see Warnings and Precautions (5.7)]
- Hypogammaglobulinemia [see Warnings and Precautions (5.8)]:

6.1 Clinical Trials Experience

Because clinical trials are conducted under widely varying conditions, adverse reaction rates observed in the clinical trials of a drug cannot be directly compared to rates in the clinical trials of another drug and may not reflect the rates observed in practice.

Pediatric and Young Adult r/r B-cell Acute Lymphoblastic Leukemia (ALL) (up to 25 years of age)

Based on a recommended dose which was weight-based, all 79 patients in the ELIANA study (Study 1) received a single intravenous dose of KYMRIAH [see Clinical Studies (14.1)]. The most common adverse reactions (> 20%) were cytokine release syndrome (77%), infections-pathogen unspecified (57%), hypogammaglobulinemia (53%), fever (42%), decreased appetite (38%), viral infectious disorders (38%), headache (35%), febrile neutropenia (34%), hemorrhage (32%), musculoskeletal pain (32%), vomiting (32%), encephalopathy (30%), bacterial infectious disorders (29%), diarrhea (29%), hypotension (29%), cough (27%), nausea (27%), pain (25%), hypoxia (25%), tachycardia (24%), edema (23%), fatigue (23%), and acute kidney injury (22%). The adverse reactions with greater or equal to 10% incidence for any Grade are summarized in Table 3.

Table 3. Selected adverse reactions any time after infusion (≥ 10%). Following treatment with Kymriah in pediatric and young adult r/r b-cell ALL (N = 68). Please note that the ***italics*** text in Table 4 and the footnotes to Table 4 are used in the FDA package insert.

Adverse reaction	All grades (%)	Grades 3 or higher (%)
Blood and lymphatic system disorders:		
Febrile Neutropenia	37	37
Cardiac disorders		
Tachycardia[a]	26	4
Gastrointestinal disorders:		
Nausea	26	3
Diarrhea	26	1
Vomiting	26	1
Constipation	18	0
Abdominal pain[b]	16	3
General disorders and administration site conditions:		
Pyrexia	40	15
Fatigue[c]	25	0
Edema[d]	21	1
Chills	10	0
Pain[e]	18	3

Infections and infestations:		
Infections - pathogen unspecified	41	16
Viral infectious disorders	26	18
Bacterial infectious disorders	19	13
Fungal infectious disorders	13	7
Investigations:		
International normalized ratio increased	13	0
Metabolism and nutrition disorders:		
Decreased appetite	37	15
Fluid overload	10	7
Musculoskeletal and connective tissue disorders:		
Myalgia	15	0
Arthralgia	12	1
Back pain	10	3
Nervous system disorders:		

Headache[g]	37	3
Encephalopathy[h]	34	10
Psychiatric disorders:		
Delirium[i]	21	4
Anxiety	13	3
Sleep disorders[j]	10	0
Respiratory, thoracic and mediastinal disorders:		
Hypoxia	24	18
Cough[l]	21	0
Dyspnea[m]	16	12
Pulmonary edema	16	10
Tachypnea	12	6
Pleural effusion	10	4
Nasal congestion	10	0
Skin and subcutaneous tissue disorders:		
Rash[n]	16	1
Vascular disorders:		
Hypotension	31	22
Hypertension	19	6

[a] *Tachycardia includes tachycardia and sinus tachycardia.*

[b] *Abdominal pain includes abdominal pain, abdominal pain upper.*

[c] *Fatigue includes fatigue and malaise.*

[d] *Edema includes face edema, generalised edema, localised edema, edema peripheral.*

[e] *Pain includes pain and pain in the extremity.*

[f]*Hypogammaglobulinemia includes hypogammaglobulinemia, immunoglobulins decreased, blood immunoglobulin G decreased, blood immunoglobulin A decreased, blood immunoglobulin M decreased.*

[g]*Headache includes headache and migraine.*

[h]*Encephalopathy includes encephalopathy, cognitive disorder, confusional state, depressed level of consciousness, disturbance in attention, lethargy, mental status changes, somnolence, and automatism.*

[i]*Delirium includes delirium, agitation, hallucination, hallucination visual, irritability, restlessness.*

[j]*Sleep disorders includes sleep disorder, insomnia and nightmare.*

[k]*Acute kidney injury includes acute kidney injury, anuria, azotemia, renal failure, renal tubular dysfunction, renal tubular necrosis, and blood creatinine increased.*

[l]*Cough includes cough and productive cough.*

[m]*Dyspnea includes dyspnea and respiratory distress, respiratory failure.*

[n]*Rash includes rash, rash maculo-papular, rash papular, and rash pruritic.*

Additional important adverse reactions that did not meet the threshold criteria for inclusion in Table 4 were:

Blood and lymphatic system disorders: disseminated intravascular coagulation (9%); histiocytosis lymphocytic hemophagocytosis (7%); coagulopathy (6%); Grade 3 and Grade 4 hypofibrinogenemia with Grade 3 and 4 CRS (16%).

Cardiac disorders: cardiac arrest (4%), cardiac failure (7%).

Gastrointestinal disorders: abdominal compartment syndrome (1%).

General disorders and administration site conditions: multiple organ dysfunction syndrome (3%).

Immune system disorders: graft-versus-host disease (1%).

Investigations: activated partial thromboplastin time prolonged (6%).

Nervous system: tremor (9%), dizziness (6%), seizure (3%), speech disorders[a] (3%), motor dysfunction[b] including muscle spasms (1%)

Respiratory, thoracic, and mediastinal disorders: respiratory distress (6%), respiratory failure (6%), acute respiratory distress syndrome (4%), oropharyngeal pain (6%).

Metabolism and nutrition disorders: tumor lysis syndrome (6%).

Vascular disorders: capillary leak syndrome (3%), thrombosis (3%)

Eye disorders: visual impairment (3%)

[a]Speech disorder includes aphasia and dysarthria. [b]Motor dysfunction includes muscle spasms.

*[Some of the above disorders are described further below: This information is **not** included in the FDA package insert and thus they are placed in parentheses and written in italics.*

*[**Hemophagocytic lymphohistiocytosis** (HLH), also known as haemophagocytic lymphohistiocytosis (British spelling), and hemophagocytic or haemophagocytic syndrome, is an uncommon hematologic disorder seen more often in children than in adults. It is a life-threatening disease of severe hyperinflammation caused by uncontrolled proliferation of activated lymphocytes and macrophages, characterised by proliferation of morphologically benign lymphocytes and macrophages that secrete high amounts of inflammatory cytokines. It is classified as one of the cytokine storm syndromes. There are inherited and non-inherited (acquired) causes of hemophagocytic lymphohistiocytosis (HLH).*

Figure 15. Light microscopic image of bone marrow showing stromal macrophages containing numerous red blood cells in their cytoplasm.

This image is by Jon salisbury at English Wikipedia - Transferred from en.wikipedia to Commons. Public Domain, https://commons.wikimedia.org/w/index.php?curid=11557969; https://en.wikipedia.org/wiki/Hemophagocytic_lymphohistiocytosis#/media/File:Haemophagocytic_lymphohistiocytosis_Bone_marrow.JPG. This work has been released into the public domain by its author, Jon salisbury at English Wikipedia. No changes were made to this image).

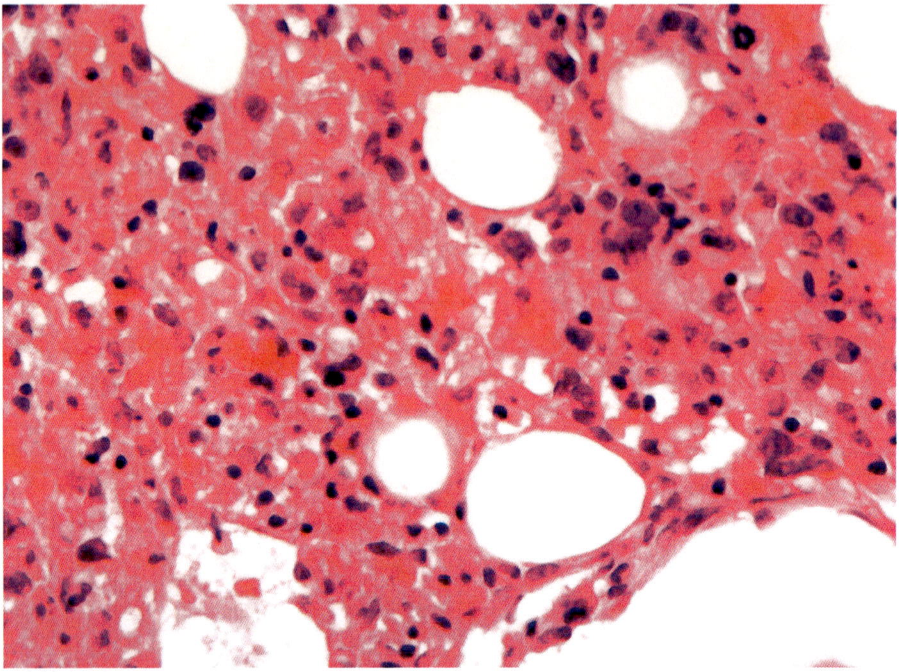

(Hypogammaglobulinemia

Hypogammaglobulinemia is a situation with the immune system in which not enough gamma globulins are produced in the blood. This results in a lower antibody count, which impairs the immune system, increasing risk of infection. Hypogammaglobulinemia may result from a variety of primary genetic immune system defects, such as common variable immunodeficiency, or it may be caused by secondary effects such as medication, blood cancer, or poor nutrition, or loss of gamma globulins in urine, as in nonselective glomerular proteinuria. Patients with hypogammaglobulinemia have reduced immune function; important considerations include avoiding use of live vaccines, and take precautionary measures when traveling to regions with endemic disease or poor sanitation such as receiving immunizations, taking antibiotics abroad, drinking only safe or boiled water, arranging appropriate medical cover in advance of travel, and ensuring continuation of any immunoglobulin infusions needed).

(Capillary leak syndrome.

Capillary leak syndrome is characterized by the escape of blood plasma through capillary walls, from the blood circulatory system to surrounding tissues, muscle compartments, organs or body cavities. It is a phenomenon most commonly witnessed in sepsis, and less frequently in autoimmune diseases, ***differentiation syndrome***, ***engraftment syndrome***, *hemophagocytic lymphohistiocytosis [see above], the* ***ovarian hyperstimulation syndrome***, *viral hemorrhagic fevers, and snakebite and ricin poisoning. Pharmaceuticals, including the chemotherapy medications gemcitabine and tagraxofusp, as well as certain interleukins and monoclonal antibodies, can also cause capillary leaks. These conditions and factors are sources of secondary capillary leak syndrome.*

(Differentiation syndrome

Differentiation syndrome, formerly known as Retinoic acid syndrome (RAS), is a potentially life-threatening complication observed in people with acute promyelocytic leukemia (APML) and first thought to be specifically associated with all-trans retinoic acid (ATRA) (also known as tretinoin) treatment. Subsequently, so-called RAS was recognized in APML patients who had been treated with another highly efficacious drug, arsenic trioxide, and yet did not appear in patients treated with tretinoin for other disorders. These facts and others support the notion that RAS depends on the presence of the malignant promyelocytes. This has led to the growing deprecation of the term 'retinoic acid syndrome' and to an increasing use of the term differentiation syndrome to signify this APML treatment complication.

(Engraftment syndrome

Engraftment syndrome (ES) is an early complication of hematopoietic stem cell transplantation (HSCT) that occurs around neutrophil engraftment time and is attributed to the sudden cytokine discharge associated with robust engraftment of transplanted cells. The secreted cytokines cause a clinical picture suggestive of an exaggerated inflammatory response. This complication has been described both in autologous and allogeneic transplantation.
The diagnostic clinical features include the presence of two or more of the following symptoms usually 96 hours before neutrophil engraftment time: 1. fever of unknown origin (38.0-38.5 °C) with no detectable infectious agent or other cause, 2. erythematous skin rash not related to drug reactions or viral infection (usually covering >25% of the body surface), 3. weight gain of 2.5-5% (above baseline of admission) and albumin drop to 90% of pretransplant levels, and 4. pulmonary symptoms with dyspnea, hypoxia and pulmonary infiltrates on a chest X-ray (excluding infection, thromboembolism, pulmonary hemorrhage, fluid overload, or cardiac causes). Though hepatic dysfunction, renal insufficiency and

transient encephalopathy have been described in adults, they have not been reported as common findings in pediatric practice.

Risk Factors include;1. High cell doses infused on day 0, 2. Prompt increase in white blood cell (WBC) counts, 3. Autologous peripheral blood as stem cell source, and 4. Autoimmune disease as an underlying condition.

Differential diagnosis and early recognition are particularly important since corticosteroids have a critical role in the reversal of symptoms and management of the condition.

The prognosis is usually good with early corticosteroid use, and complete resolution is seen in 1-5 days in >80% of cases. Otherwise, this complication occasionally may lead to increased morbidity and mortality if not managed appropriately and timely. ES is associated with increased length of hospitalization. It may be problematic since it can resemble cutaneous acute graft-versus-host disease (aGvHD) or be complicated by capillary leak syndrome and noncardiogenic pulmonary edema. Rarely, ES can mimic aGvHD by affecting the liver and gastrointestinal tract. It has been shown that patients who develop ES receive empirical antifungal therapy more frequently than patients who do not, most likely due to persistent fever. Patients undergoing autologous HSCT for multiple sclerosis who develop ES may experience transient worsening of neurological symptoms. In pediatric patients, ES is also associated with increased transfusion requirements, need for parenteral nutrition and increased risk of critical care requirement

Corticosteroids also have a role in the prevention of ES.

(Multiple organ dysfunction syndrome

Multiple dysfunction syndrome is the presence of altered organ function in acutely ill patients such that homeostasis cannot be maintained without intervention. It usually involves two or more organ systems. It calls for an immediate intervention. Although Irwin and Rippe cautioned in 2005 that the use of "multiple organ failure" or "multisystem organ failure" should be avoided, both Harrison's (2015) and Cecil's (2012) medical textbooks still use the terms "multi-organ failure" and "multiple organ failure" in several chapters and do not use "multiple organ dysfunction syndrome" at all.

The condition results from infection, injury (accident, surgery), hypoperfusion and hypermetabolism. The primary cause triggers an uncontrolled inflammatory response.

Sepsis is the most common cause of multiple organ dysfunction syndrome and may result in septic shock. In the absence of infection, a sepsis-like disorder is termed systemic inflammatory response syndrome (SIRS). Both SIRS and sepsis could ultimately progress to multiple organ dysfunction syndrome. However, in one-third of the patients no primary focus can be found. Multiple organ dysfunction syndrome is well established as the final stage of a continuum: SIRS + infection → sepsis → severe sepsis → Multiple organ dysfunction syndrome.

At present, there is no drug or device that can reverse organ failure that has been judged by the health care team to be medically and/or surgically irreversible (organ function can recover, at least to a degree, in patients whose organs are very dysfunctional, where the patient has not died, and some organs, like the liver or the skin, can regenerate better than others),- with the possible exception of single or multiple organ transplants or the use of artificial organs or organ parts, in certain candidates in specific situations. Therapy, therefore, is usually mostly limited to supportive care, i.e. safeguarding hemodynamics, and respiration. Maintaining adequate tissue oxygenation is a principal target. Starting enteral nutrition within 36 hours of admission to an intensive care unit has reduced infectious complications.

Mortality, though it has lessened to a limited degree, at least in high income countries with timely access to initial and tertiary care, varies where the chance of survival is diminished as the number of organs involved increases. Mortality in MODS from septic shock (which itself has a mortality of 25-50%), and from multiple traumas, especially if not rapidly treated, appear to be especially severe. If more than one organ system is affected, the mortality rate is higher, and this is especially the case when five or more systems or organs are affected. Old age is a risk factor in and of itself, and immunocompromised patients, such as with cancer or HIV/AIDS or recipients of organ transplants, are at risk. Earlier and aggressive treatment, the use of experimental treatments, or at least modern tools such as ventilators, ECMO, dialysis, bypass, and transplantation, especially at a trauma center, may improve outcomes in certain cases, but this depends in part on speedy and affordable access to high-quality care. Measurements of lactate, cytokines, albumin and other proteins, urea, blood oxygen and carbon dioxide levels, insulin, and blood sugar, adequate hydration, constant monitoring of vital signs, good communication within and between facilities and staff, and adequate staffing, training, and charting are important in MODS.

(Tumor lysis syndrome

Tumor lysis syndrome (TLS) is a group of metabolic abnormalities that can occur as a complication from the treatment of cancer, where large amounts of tumor cells are lysed from the treatment, releasing their contents into the bloodstream. This occurs most commonly after the treatment of lymphomas and leukemias and in particular when treating non-Hodgkin's lymphoma (NHL), acute myeloid leukemia (AML), and acute lymphoblastic leukemia. This is a potentially fatal complication and patients at increased risk for TLS should be closely monitored while receiving chemotherapy and should receive preventive measures and treatments TLS can also occur on its own (while not being treated with chemotherapy) although this is less common.

Tumor lysis syndrome is characterized by hyperkalemia, hyperphosphatemia, hypocalcemia), hyperuricemia and higher than normal levels of blood urea nitrogen (BUN). These changes in blood electrolytes and metabolites are a result of the release of cellular contents of dying cells into the bloodstream. In this respect, TLS is analogous to rhabdomyolysis, with comparable mechanism and blood chemistry effects but with a different cause. In TLS, the breakdown occurs after cytotoxic therapy or from cancers with high cell turnover and tumor proliferation rates. The metabolic abnormalities seen in tumor lysis syndrome can ultimately result in serious complications such as acute uric acid nephropathy, acute kidney failure, seizures, cardiac arrhythmias, and death.

It can be prevented by prophylactically ensuring good renal output with administration of intravenous fluids and a loop diuretic together with rasburicase to help clear uric acid from the blood. Mild hyperkalemia without symptoms can be treated with a loop diuretic and sodium polystirene, while a temporizing agent such as rapid acting insulin (in conjunction with glucose) and an agent to stabilize cardiac membranes such as calcium carbonate may be given in cases of severe hyperkalemia. For symptoms due to hypocalcemia (e.g. seizures) patients can be treated with calcium gluconate. Tumor lysis patients may ultimately also require renal replacement therapy such as through hemodialysis if indicated.

(Graft-versus-host disease.

Graft-versus-host disease (GvHD) is a syndrome, characterized by inflammation in different organs, most commonly associated with hematopoietic stem cell transplants. T cells of the donor's immune system which remain within the donated tissue (the graft) recognize the recipient (the host) as foreign (non-self). The T cells present within the transplanted tissue then attack the recipient's body's cells, which leads to GvHD. This should not be confused with a transplant rejection, which occurs when the immune system of the transplant recipient rejects the transplanted tissue. GvHD occurs when the donor's immune system's T cells reject the recipient. GvHD can also occur after a blood transfusion if the blood products used have not been irradiated or treated with an approved pathogen reduction system).

(Ovarian hyperstimulation syndrome.

Ovarian hyperstimulation syndrome (OHSS) is a medical condition that can occur in some women who take fertility medication to stimulate egg growth, and in other women in very rare cases. Most cases are mild, but rarely the condition is severe and can lead to serious illness or death. Symptoms can be mild, moderate, or severe. Mild symptoms include abdominal bloating and feeling of fullness, nausea, diarrhea, and slight weight gain. Moderate symptoms include excessive weight gain (weight gain of greater than 2 pounds per day), increased abdominal girth, vomiting, diarrhea, darker urine, decreased urine output, excessive thirst, and skin and/or hair feeling dry (in addition to mild symptoms). Severe symptoms are fullness/bloating above the waist, shortness of breath, pleural effusion, urination significantly darker or has ceased, calf and chest pains, marked abdominal bloating or distention, and lower abdominal pains (in addition to mild and moderate symptoms).

The central feature of clinically significant OHSS is the development of vascular hyperpermeability and the resulting shift of fluids into the third space. As hCG causes the ovary to undergo extensive luteinization, large amounts of estrogens, progesterone, and local cytokines are released. It is almost certain that vascular endothelial growth factor (VEGF) is a key substance that induces vascular hyperpermeability, making local capillaries "leaky", leading to a shift of fluids from the intravascular system to the abdominal and pleural cavity. Supraphysiologic production of VEGF from many follicles under the prolonged effect of hCG appears to be the specific key process underlying OHSS. Thus, while the woman accumulates fluid in the third space, primarily in the form of ascites, she actually becomes hypovolemic and is at risk for respiratory, circulatory (such as arterial thromboembolism since blood is now thicker), and renal problems. Women who are pregnant sustain the ovarian luteinization process through the production of hCG)].

Laboratory abnormalities

Table 4. Selected other laboratory abnormalities worsening (>10%) from baseline grade 0-2 to grade 3 – 4 following treatment with KYMRIAH in pediatric and young adult patients with r/r B cell ALL based on CTCAE[a] (N = 68).

Laboratory abnormality	**Grade 3-4 (%)**
Increased aspartate transaminase	28
Hypokalemia	27
Increased Alanine Aminotransferase	21
Increased bilirubin	21

Hypophosphatemia	19
Hyperglycemia	11

All patients experienced neutropenia, anemia and thrombocytopenia. See Table 5 for the incidences of ≥ Grade 3 prolonged thrombocytopenia and prolonged neutropenia in responding patients.

[C]TCAE = Common Terminology Criteria for Adverse Events version 4.03

Table 5. Prolonged cytopenias following treatment with KYMRIAH in pediatric and young adult patients with r/r B cell ALL.

Prolonged cytopenia	N = 52 (%) Day 28	N = 52 (%) Day 56
Prolonged neutropenia[a]	40	17
Prolonged thrombocytopenia[a]	27	12

[a] ≥ Grade 3 observed within 14 days after Day 28 or Day 56 in responding patients

6.2 Postmarketing Experience

The following adverse reaction has been identified during postapproval use of KYMRIAH. Because this reaction is reported voluntarily from a population of uncertain size, it is not always possible to reliably estimate its frequency or establish a causal relationship to drug exposure.

- Anaphylactic reaction

6.3. Immunogenicity

In clinical studies, humoral immunogenicity of KYMRIAH was measured by determination of anti-murine CAR19 antibodies (anti-mCAR19) in serum pre- and post-administration. The majority of patients, 86% in ELIANA (Study 1) and 91.4% in JULIET (Study 2) tested positive for pre-dose anti-mCAR19 antibodies prior to KYMRIAH infusion; Treatment induced anti-mCAR19 antibodies were detected in 5% of the patients in JULIET. However, the pre-existing and treatment-induced antibodies were not associated with an impact on clinical response and did not have an impact on the initial expansion and persistence of KYMRIAH. Persistence of KYMRIAH was similar between patients with positive post-infusion anti-mCAR19 antibodies compared with patients with negative post-infusion anti-mCAR19 antibodies. There is no evidence that the presence of pre-existing and treatment-induced anti-mCAR19 antibodies impact the safety or effectiveness of KYMRIAH.

7. DRUG INTERACTIONS

HIV and the lentivirus used to make KYMRIAH have limited, short spans of identical genetic material (RNA). Therefore, some commercial HIV nucleic acid test (NATs) tests may yield false-positive results in patients who have received KYMRIAH.

USE IN SPECIFIC POPULATIONS

Pregnancy

Risk summary

There are no available data with KYMRIAH use in pregnant women. No animal reproductive and developmental toxicity studies have been conducted with KYMRIAH to assess whether it can cause fetal harm when administered to a pregnant woman. It is not known if KYMRIAH has the potential to be transferred to the fetus. Based on the mechanism of action, if the transduced cells cross the placenta, they may cause fetal toxicity, including B-cell lymphocytopenia. Therefore, KYMRIAH is not recommended for women who are pregnant, and pregnancy after KYMRIAH administration should be discussed with the treating physician. Report pregnancies to Novartis Pharmaceuticals Corporation at 1-888-669-6682. In the U.S. general population, the estimated background risk of major birth defects and miscarriage in clinically recognized pregnancies is 2%-4% and 15%-20%, respectively.

Lactation

Risk summary

There is no information regarding the presence of KYMRIAH in human milk, the effect on the breastfed infant, and the effects on milk production. The developmental and health benefits of breastfeeding should be considered along with the mother's clinical need for KYMRIAH and any potential adverse effects on the breastfed infant from KYMRIAH or from the underlying maternal condition.

8.3. Females and Males of Reproductive Potential

Pregnancy testing

Pregnancy status of females with reproductive potential should be verified. Sexually-active females of reproductive potential should have a pregnancy test prior to starting treatment with KYMRIAH.

Contraception

See the prescribing information for fludarabine and cyclophosphamide for information on the need for effective contraception in patients who receive the lymphodepleting chemotherapy. There are insufficient exposure data to provide a recommendation concerning duration of contraception following treatment with KYMRIAH.

Infertility

There are no data on the effect of KYMRIAH on fertility.

8.4. Pediatric use

The safety and efficacy of KYMRIAH have been established in pediatric patients with r/r B-cell ALL. Use of KYMRIAH is supported by a single-arm trial that included 52 pediatric patients with r/r B-cell precursor ALL in the following age groups: 33 children (age 3 years to less than 12 years) and 19 adolescents (age 12 years to less than 17 years). No differences in efficacy or safety were observed between the different age subgroups or in comparison to the young adults in the trial.

8.5. Geriatric use

The safety and effectiveness of KYMRIAH have not been established in geriatric patients with r/r B-cell ALL. Clinical studies of KYMRIAH did not include sufficient numbers of subjects aged 65 and over to determine whether they respond differently from younger subjects.

11. DESCRIPTION

KYMRIAH (tisagenlecleucel) is a CD19-directed genetically modified autologous T cell immunotherapy comprised of autologous T cells that are genetically modified using a lentiviral vector to encode an anti-CD19 chimeric antigen receptor (CAR). The CAR is comprised of a murine single-chain antibody fragment (scFv) specific for CD19, followed by a CD8 hinge and transmembrane region that is fused to the intracellular signaling domains for 4-1BB (CD137) and CD3 zeta.

KYMRIAH is prepared from the patient's peripheral blood mononuclear cells, which are obtained via a standard leukapheresis procedure. The mononuclear cells are enriched for T cells, then transduced with the lentiviral vector containing the anti-CD19 CAR transgene, and activated with anti-CD3/CD28 antibody coated beads. The transduced T cells are expanded in cell culture, washed, and formulated into a suspension, which then is cryopreserved. The product must pass a sterility test before release for shipping as a frozen suspension in a patient-specific infusion bag(s). The product is thawed prior to administration [see Dosage and Administration (2.3), How Supplied/Storage and Handling (16)].

The thawed product is a colorless to slightly yellow suspension of cells. In addition to T cells, other cell populations, including monocytes, NK cells, and B-cells, may be present. The formulation contains 31.25% (v/v) of Plasma-Lyte A, 31.25% (v/v) of 5% Dextrose/0.45% sodium chloride, 10% Dextran 40 (LMD)/5% Dextrose, 20% (v/v) of 25% Human Serum Albumin (HSA), and 7.5% (v/v) Cryoserv® dimethylsulfoxide (DMSO).

Pediatric and Young Adult r/r B-cell ALL

A single dose of KYMRIAH may contain up to 2.5 x 10^8 CAR-positive viable T cells provided in one to three patient-specific infusion bag(s). Based on the patient's weight reported at the time of leukapheresis, one of two possible dose ranges will be prepared for the patient:

• For patients 50 kg or less: 0.2 to 5.0 x 10^6 CAR-positive viable T cells per kg body weight.

• For patients above 50 kg: 0.1 to 2.5 x 10^8 CAR-positive viable T cells.

12. CLINICAL PHARMACOLOGY

12.1. Mechanism of Action

KYMRIAH is a CD19-directed genetically modified autologous T cell immunotherapy which involves reprogramming a patient's own T cells with a transgene encoding a chimeric antigen receptor (CAR) to identify and eliminate CD19-expressing malignant and normal cells. The CAR is comprised of a murine single-chain antibody fragment which recognizes CD19 and is fused to intracellular signalling domains from 4-1BB (CD137) and CD3 zeta. The CD3 zeta component is critical for initiating T cell activation and antitumor activity, while 4-1BB enhances the expansion and persistence of KYMRIAH. Upon binding to CD19-expressing cells, the CAR transmits a signal to promote T cell expansion, activation, target cell elimination, and persistence of the KYMRIAH cells.

12.2 Pharmacodynamics

Due to the on-target effect of KYMRIAH, a period of B-cell aplasia is expected. Among evaluable pediatric and young adult r/r B-cell ALL patients with an ongoing response at Month 24, 33% had no detectable B cells at baseline prior to infusion. At Month 24, 88% had no detectable B cells.

12.3 Pharmacokinetics/Cellular Kinetics

Following infusion, KYMRIAH exhibited an initial rapid expansion followed by a bi-exponential decline in pediatric and young adult r/r B-cell acute lymphoblastic leukemia (ALL) patients.

Description of Pharmacokinetics in Pediatric and Young Adult r/r B-cell ALL (up to 25 years of age)

The Cmax and AUC 0-28d were similar between CR/CRi patients compared with non-responding (NR) patients. KYMRIAH was present in the blood as well as bone marrow and was measurable beyond 2 years. Blood to bone marrow partitioning suggested that KYMRIAH distribution in bone marrow was 44% of that present in blood at Day 28 while at Months 3 and 6 KYMRIAH distributed at 67% and 69%, respectively, indicating high distribution to bone marrow. Children < 10 years and between 10-18 years of age had similar- to 1.7-fold higher Cmax and AUC 0-28d than adults. Due to small sample size and high variability, it is difficult to assess the impact of age on the pharmacokinetics of KYMRIAH.

Tocilizumab and Corticosteroid used for CRS Management

Some patients required tocilizumab and corticosteroids for the management of CRS. KYMRIAH continues to expand and persist following treatment as per the CRS management algorithm (see Table 1). Patients who have higher expansion tended to have higher CRS Grades [see Warnings and Precautions (5.1)]. Pediatric and young adult r/r B-cell ALL patients (N = 28) treated with tocilizumab had 298% and 183% higher KYMRIAH AUC 0-28d and Cmax, respectively, as compared to patients (N = 46) who did not receive tocilizumab. In addition, patients who received corticosteroids for CRS management (N=17) had 280% higher AUC 0-28d compared with patients who did not receive corticosteroids (N = 31).

13. NONCLINICAL TOXICOLOGY

13.1. Carcinogenesis, Mutagenesis, Impairment of Fertility

Genotoxicity assays and carcinogenicity assessment in rodent models were not performed for KYMRIAH. In vitro expansion studies with transduced T cells (KYMRIAH) from healthy donors and patients showed no evidence for transformation and/or immortalization of T cells. In vivo studies in immunocompromised mice did not show signs of abnormal cell growth or signs of clonal cell expansion for up to 7 months after cell injection. A genomic insertion site analysis was performed on KYMRIAH products from 14 individual donors (12 patients and 2 healthy volunteers). There was no evidence for preferential integration near genes of concern, or preferential outgrowth of cells harboring integration sites of concern. No studies on the effects of KYMRIAH on fertility have been conducted.

14. CLINICAL STUDIES

14.1. Relapsed or refractory (r/r) B-cell acute lymphoblastic leukemia (ALL)

The efficacy of KYMRIAH in pediatric and young adults with r/r B-cell precursor ALL was evaluated in an open-label, multicenter single-arm trial (ELIANA, NCT02228096). In total, 107 patients were screened,

88 were enrolled, 68 were treated, and 63 were evaluable for efficacy. Nine percent of the enrolled patients did not receive the product due to manufacturing failure. The 63 evaluable patients included 35 males and 28 females of median age 12 years (range: 3-23 years). Seventy-three percent of patients were White, 10% were Asian, and 17% were of other races. Six (10%) had primary refractory disease, 30 (48%) had one prior stem cell transplant, 5 patients (8%) had two stem cell transplants. Treatment consisted of lymphodepleting chemotherapy (fludarabine 30 mg/m^2 daily for 4 days and cyclophosphamide 500 mg/m^2 daily for 2 days) followed by a single dose of KYMRIAH. Of the 22 patients who had a WBC count < 1000/μL, 20 received lymphodepleting chemotherapy prior to KYMRIAH while 2 received KYMRIAH infusion without lymphodepleting chemotherapy. Fifty-three patients received bridging chemotherapy between time of enrollment and lymphodepleting chemotherapy. The efficacy of KYMRIAH was established on the basis of complete remission (CR) within 3 months after infusion, the duration of CR, and proportion of patients with CR and minimal residual disease (MRD) < 0.01% by flow cytometry (MRD-negative) are shown in Table 10). Among the 63 infused patients, 52 (83%) achieved CR/CRi, all of which were minimal residual disease (MRD)-negative. With a median follow-up of 4.8 months from response, the median duration of CR/CRi was not reached (range: 1.2 to 14.1+ months). Median time to onset of CR/CRi was 29 days with onset of CR/CRi between 26 and 31 days for 50/52 (96%) responders. The stem cell transplantation rate among those who achieved CR/CRi was 12% (6/52).

Table 10. Efficacy results in pediatric and young adult patients with r/r B-cell ALL Results. N = 63.

Results	**N = 63**
CR/Cri[1,2]	52 (83%)
95% CI	71%, 91%
	p<0.0001
CR[3]	40 (63%)
Cri[4]	12 (19%)
CR or CRi with MRD-negative bone marrow[5,6]	52 (83%)
95% CI	71%, 91%
	p<0.0001
Duration of remission[7]	N = 52
Median (months)	Not reached
95% CI	7.5, Not reached[8]

[1]CR/CRi was calculated based on all patients who received KYMRIAH and completed at least 3 months follow-up, or discontinued earlier prior to the data cut-off. Requires remission status to be maintained for at least 28 days without clinical evidence of relapse.

[2]The null hypothesis of CR/CRi less than or equal to 20% was rejected.

[3]CR (complete remission) was defined as less than 5% of blasts in the bone marrow, no evidence of extramedullary disease, and full recovery of peripheral blood counts (platelets greater than 100,000/microliter and absolute neutrophil counts [ANC] greater than 1,000/microliter) without blood transfusion.

[4]CRi (complete remission with incomplete blood count recovery) was defined as less than 5% of blasts in the bone marrow, no evidence of extramedullary disease, and without full recovery of peripheral blood counts with or without blood transfusion. [5]MRD (minimal residual disease) negative was defined as MRD by flow cytometry less than 0.01%.

[6]The null hypothesis of MRD-negative remission rate less than or equal to 15% was rejected.

[7]DOR (duration of remission) was defined as time since onset of CR or CRi to relapse or death due to underlying cancer, whichever is earlier, censoring for new cancer therapy including stem cell transplantation (N = 52).

[8]Not estimable.

15. REFERENCES

1. Porter DL, Hwang WT, Frey N, et al (2015). Chimeric antigen receptor T cells persist and induce sustained remissions in relapsed refractory chronic lymphocytic leukemia (Table S4A). Sci. Transl Med; 7(303):303ra139. DOI: 10.1126/scitranslmed.aac5415.

2. Lee DW, Gardner R, Porter DL, et al (2014). Current concepts in the diagnosis and management of cytokine release syndrome. Blood; 124(2):188-95.

3. Lee DW, Santomasso BD, Locke FL, et al (2019) ASTCT Consensus Grading for Cytokine Release Syndrome and Neurologic Toxicity Associated with Immune Effector Cells. Biol Blood Marrow Transplant; 25(4):625-38.

4. Santomosso BD, Nastoupil LJ, Adkins S, et al (2021) Management of Immune-Related Adverse Events in Patients Treated With Chimeric Antigen Receptor T-Cell Therapy: ASCO Guideline. J Clin Oncol; 39(35):3978-92.

16. HOW SUPPLIED/STORAGE AND HANDLING

KYMRIAH is supplied as a frozen suspension of genetically modified autologous T cells in an infusion bag(s) labeled for the specific recipient. KYMRIAH is shipped directly to the cell lab associated with the infusion center in a liquid nitrogen Dewar. Product and patient-specific labels are located inside the Dewar.

• Confirm patient identity upon receipt.Store infusion bag(s) in a temperature-monitored system less than or equal to minus 120°C, e.g., in the vapor phase of liquid nitrogen.

• Use closed, break-proof, leak-proof containers when transporting infusion bags within the facility.

• Thaw KYMRIAH prior to infusion [see Dosage and Administration (2)].

[Author's comment:

Similarities between tisangelecleucel/Kymriah and brexucabtagene/Tecartus are that both target CD19.

Differences between them are that

1. *Kymriah is approved for children and young adults with r/r B cell ALL, Tescartus is approved for adults with r/r B cell ALL*
2. *The co-stimulatory domains used in Kymriah are CD137 and CD3 zeta, whereas those used in Tecartus are CD28 and CD3 zeta.*

Many other aspects of the three drugs are similar – for example, their toxicities.

The FDA label for each is available online and is in the public domain.

Please note that this book deals only with the FDA approval of TECARTUS for people with refractory acute lymphoblastic leukemia, and not with its other FDA approval for people with refractory Mantle Cell Lymphoma].

14. BREXUCABTAGENE/TECARTUS

BOXED WARNING: CYTOKINE RELEASE SYNDROME and NEUROLOGIC TOXICITIES

- **Cytokine release syndrome (CRS), including life-threatening reactions, occurred in patients receiving TECARTUS. Do not administer TECARTUS to patients with active infection or inflammatory disorders. Treat severe or life-threatening CRS with tocilizumab or tocilizumab and corticosteroids**
- **Neurologic toxicities, including life-threatening reactions, occurred in patients receiving TECARTUS, including concurrently with CRS or after CRS resolution. Monitor for neurologic toxicities after treatment with TECARTUS. Provide supportive care and/or corticosteroids, as needed.**
- **TECARTUS is available only through a restricted program under a Risk Evaluation and Mitigation Strategy (REMS) called the YESCARTA and TECARTUS REMS Program.**

12.1. Mechanism of action

TECARTUS, a CD19-directed genetically modified autologous T cell immunotherapy, binds to CD19-expressing cancer cells and normal B cells. Studies demonstrated that following anti-CD19 CAR T cell engagement with CD19-expressing target cells, the CD28 and CD3 zeta co-stimulatory domains activate downstream signaling cascades that lead to T cell activation, proliferation, acquisition of effector functions, and secretion of inflammatory cytokines and chemokines. This sequence of events leads to killing of CD19- expressing cells.

FULL PRESCRIBING INFORMATION: CONTENTS*

WARNING: CYTOKINE RELEASE SYNDROME AND NEUROLOGIC TOXICITIES (see Boxed Warning above)

* Sections or subsections omitted from the full Prescribing Information are not listed.

1. INDICATIONS AND USAGE

TECARTUS is a CD19-directed genetically modified autologous T cell immunotherapy indicated for the treatment of

1.2. B cell acute lymphoblastic leukemia

Adult patients with relapsed or refractory B-cell precursor acute lymphoblastic leukemia (ALL).

2 DOSAGE AND ADMINISTRATION

For autologous use only. For intravenous use only.

Each single infusion bag of TECARTUS contains a suspension of chimeric antigen receptor (CAR)-positive T cells in approximately 68 mL.

2.1. Dose

Recommended Dosage for ALL

The target dose is 1 × 10^6 CAR-positive viable T cells per kg body weight, with a maximum of 1 × 10^8 CAR- positive viable T cells.

ADMINISTRATION

TECARTUS is for autologous use only. The patient's identity must match the patient identifiers on the TECARTUS cassette and infusion bag. Do not infuse TECARTUS if the information on the patient-specific label does not match the intended patient. *Preparing the patient for TECARTUS Infusion*

Confirm availability of TECARTUS prior to starting the lymphodepleting chemotherapy regimen.

Pre-treatment

• ALL: administer a lymphodepleting chemotherapy regimen of fludarabine 25 mg/m^2 intravenously over 30 minutes on the fourth, third, and second day and administer cyclophosphamide 900 mg/m^2 over 60 minutes on the second day before infusion of TECARTUS.

Premedication

• Premedicate with acetaminophen and diphenhydramine or another H1-antihistamine approximately 30 to 60 minutes prior to TECARTUS infusion.

• Avoid prophylactic use of systemic corticosteroids as it may interfere with the activity of TECARTUS.

Preparation of TECARTUS for infusion

Coordinate the timing of TECARTUS thaw and infusion. Confirm the infusion time in advance, and adjust the start time of TECARTUS thaw such that TECARTUS will be available for infusion when the patient is ready.

• Confirm patient identity

Prior to TECARTUS preparation, match the patient's identity with the patient identifiers on the TECARTUS cassette.

• Do not remove the TECARTUS infusion bag from the cassette if the patient information on the cassette label does not match the intended patient.

• Once patient identity is confirmed, remove the TECARTUS infusion bag from the cassette and check that the patient information on the cassette label matches the patient information on the bag label.

• Inspect the infusion bag for any breaches of container integrity such as breaks or cracks before thawing. If the bag is compromised, follow the local guidelines (or call Kite at 1-844-454-KITE).

• Place the infusion bag inside a second sterile bag per local guidelines.

• Thaw the infusion bag at approximately 37°C using either a water bath or dry-thaw method until there is no visible ice in the infusion bag.

• Gently mix the contents of the bag to disperse clumps of cellular material. If visible cell clumps remain, continue to gently mix the contents of the bag. Small clumps of cellular material should disperse with gentle manual mixing. Do not wash, spin down, and/or re-suspend TECARTUS in new media prior to infusion.

• Once thawed, TECARTUS should be administered within 30 minutes but may be stored at room temperature (20°C to 25°C) for up to three hours.

Administration

• For autologous use only.

• Ensure that tocilizumab and emergency equipment are available prior to infusion and during the recovery period.

• Do NOT use a leukodepleting filter.

• Central venous access is recommended for the administration of TECARTUS.

• Confirm that the patient's identity matches the patient identifiers on the TECARTUS infusion bag.

• Prime the tubing with normal saline prior to infusion.

• Infuse the entire contents of the TECARTUS bag within 30 minutes by either gravity or a peristaltic pump. TECARTUS is stable at room temperature for up to three hours after thaw.

• Gently agitate the TECARTUS bag during infusion to prevent cell clumping.

• After the entire contents of the TECARTUS bag are infused, rinse the tubing with normal saline at the same infusion rate to ensure all product is delivered. TECARTUS contains human blood cells that are genetically modified with replication-incompetent retroviral vector. Follow universal precautions and local biosafety guidelines for handling and disposal of TECARTUS to avoid potential transmission of infectious diseases.

Monitoring

• Administer TECARTUS at a certified healthcare facility.

• Monitor patients at the certified healthcare facility daily for at least seven days for patients with MCL and at least 14 days for patients with ALL following infusion for signs and symptoms of Cytokine Release Syndrome (CRS) and neurologic events.

• Instruct patients to remain within proximity of the certified healthcare facility for at least four weeks following infusion.

2.2. Management of severe adverse reactions

Cytokine Release Syndrome

Identify CRS based on clinical presentation. Evaluate for and treat other causes of fever, hypoxia, and hypotension. If CRS is suspected, manage according to the recommendations in Table 13. *[This Table relates to Yescarta, but the recommendations are the same for Tescartus].* Patients who experience Grade 2 or higher CRS (e.g., hypotension, not responsive to fluids, or hypoxia requiring supplemental oxygenation) should be monitored with continuous cardiac telemetry and pulse oximetry. For patients experiencing severe CRS, consider performing an echocardiogram to assess cardiac function. For severe or life-threatening CRS, consider intensive care supportive therapy.

Table 1. CRS Grading and Management Guidance

CRS Grade[a]	Symptomatic treatment	Tocilizumab	Corticosteroids
Grade 1. Mild symptoms requiring symptomatic treatment only (e.g., low grade fever, fatigue, anorexia, etc.)	Exclude other causes (e.g., infection) and treat specific symptoms (e.g., with antipyretics, antiemetics, analgesics, etc.)	In patients with persistent (>3 days) or refractory fever, consider managing as Grade 2 CRS[b].	Not applicable
Grade 2. Symptoms require and respond to moderate intervention Oxygen requirement <40% or Hypotension responsive to fluids or low dose of one vasopressor or Grade 2 organ toxicity	Antipyretics, oxygen, intravenous fluids and/or low dose vasopressors as needed.	Administer tocilizumab[c] intravenously over 1 hour: − 8 mg/kg (max. 800 mg) if body weight ≥30 kg − 12 mg/kg if body weight < 30 kg If no improvement after first dose, repeat every 8 hours (limit to a maximum of 3 dosages in 24 hours period; maximum total of 4 doses).	If no improvement within 24 hours of tocilizumab, administer a daily dose of 2 mg/kg/day methylprednisolone intravenously (or equivalent) until vasopressor and oxygen no longer needed, then taper. If not improving, manage as appropriate grade below.
Grade 3. Symptoms require and respond to aggressive intervention Oxygen	High-flow oxygen Intravenous fluids, and high-dose or multiple	Per Grade 2. If not improving, consider alternative therapy[d].	Per Grade 2. If not improving, manage as Grade 4.

requirement ≥40% or Hypotension requiring high dose or multiple vasopressors or Grade 3 organ toxicity or Grade 4 transaminitis	vasopressors Treat other organ toxicities as per local guidelines		
Grade 4. Life-threatening symptoms Requirement for ventilator support or Grade 4 organ toxicity (excluding transaminitis)	Grade 4 Life-threatening symptoms Requirement for ventilator support or Grade 4 organ toxicity (excluding transaminitis)	Per Grade 2. If not improving, consider alternative therapy[d].	Administer methylprednisolone 1,000 mg intravenously one to two times per day for 3 days. If not improving, consider methylprednisolone 1,000 mg intravenously two to three times a day or alternate therapy[d]. Continue corticosteroids until improvement to Grade 1, and then taper as clinically appropriate.

References: [a]Lee et al. 2014

[b]Santomasso et al. 2021

[c]Refer to tocilizumab Prescribing Information for details.

[d]Alternative therapy includes anti-cytokine and anti-T cell therapies as per institutional policy and published guidelines such as (but not limited to) anakinra, siltuximab, ruxolitinib, cyclophosphamide, IVIG and ATG.

Neurologic Toxicity

Monitor patients for signs and symptoms of neurologic toxicities. Rule out other causes of neurologic symptoms. Patients who experience Grade 2 or higher neurologic toxicities should be monitored with continuous cardiac telemetry and pulse oximetry. Provide intensive care supportive therapy for severe or life-threatening neurologic toxicities. Consider non-sedating anti-seizure medicines (e.g., levetiracetam) for seizure prophylaxis for any Grade 2 or higher neurologic toxicities.

Table 2: Neurologic Toxicity Grading and Management Guidance

<table>
<tr><th>Neurologic Event[a]</th><th>Concurrent CRS</th><th>No Concurrent CRS</th></tr>
<tr><td>Grade 1
Examples include:
Somnolence – mild drowsiness or sleepiness
Confusion – mild disorientation
Encephalopathy – mild limiting of ADLs
Dysphasia – not impairing ability to communicate</td><td>Administer tocilizumab per Table 1 for management of Grade 1 CRS.</td><td>Supportive care.</td></tr>
<tr><td rowspan="2">Grade 2
Examples include:
Somnolence – moderate limiting instrumental ADLs
Confusion – moderate disorientation
Encephalopathy – limiting instrumental ADLs
Dysphasia moderate impairing ability to communicate spontaneously
Seizure(s)</td><td>Administer tocilizumab per Table 1 for management of Grade 2 CRS.
If not improving within 24 hours after starting tocilizumab, administer dexamethasone 10 mg intravenously every 6 hours until the event is Grade 1 or less, then taper corticosteroids.
If improving, discontinue tocilizumab.
If still not improving, manage as Grade 3.</td><td>Administer dexamethasone 10 mg intravenously every 6 hours until the event is Grade 1 or less.
If improving, taper corticosteroids.</td></tr>
<tr><td colspan="2">Consider non-sedating, anti-seizure medicines (e.g., levetiracetam) for seizure prophylaxis.</td></tr>
</table>

Neurologic Event[a]	Concurrent CRS	No Concurrent CRS
Grade 3 Examples include: Somnolence – obtundation or stupor Confusion – severe disorientation Encephalopathy – limiting self-care ADLs Dysphasia – severe receptive or expressive characteristics, impairing ability to read, write, or communicate intelligibly	Administer tocilizumab per Table 1 for management of Grade 2 CRS. In addition, administer dexamethasone 10 mg intravenously with the first dose of tocilizumab and repeat dose every 6 hours. Continue dexamethasone use until the event is Grade 1 or less, then taper corticosteroids. If improving, discontinue tocilizumab and manage as Grade 2. If still not improving, manage as Grade 4.	Administer dexamethasone 10 mg intravenously every 6 hours. Continue dexamethasone use until the event is Grade 1 or less, then taper corticosteroids. If not improving, manage as Grade 4.
	Consider non-sedating anti-seizure medicines (e.g., levetiracetam) for seizure prophylaxis.	
Grade 4 Life-threatening consequences Urgent intervention indicated Requirement for mechanical ventilation Consider cerebral edema	Administer tocilizumab per Table 1 for management of Grade 2 CRS. Administer methylprednisolone 1000 mg intravenously per day with first dose of tocilizumab and continue methylprednisolone 1000 mg intravenously per day for 2 more days. If improving, then manage as Grade 3. If not improving, consider alternate immunosuppressants.	Administer methylprednisolone 1000 mg intravenously per day for 3 days. If improving, then manage as Grade 3. If not improving, consider alternate immunosuppressants.
	Consider non-sedating anti-seizure medicines (e.g., levetiracetam) for seizure prophylaxis.	

Abbreviation: ADLs, activities of daily living.

[a]Severity based on Common Terminology Criteria for Adverse Event

3. DOSAGE FORMS AND STRENGTHS

TECARTUS is available as a cell suspension for infusion.

• ALL: A single dose of TECARTUS contains 1 x 10^6 CAR-positive viable T cells per kg of body weight [maximum of 1 x 10^8 CAR-positive viable T cells (for patients 100 kg and above)] in approximately 68 mL suspension in an infusion bag.

4. CONTRAINDICATIONS: None

5. WARNINGS AND PRECAUTIONS

5.1. Cytokine Release Syndrome (CRS) occurred in 92% (72/78) of patients with ALL, including ≥ Grade 3 (Lee grading system1) CRS in 26% of patients. Three patients with ALL had ongoing CRS events at the time of death. The median time to onset of CRS was five days (range 1 to 12 days) and the median duration of CRS was eight days (range 2 to 63 days) for patients with ALL. The incidence of CRS (first occurrence) within the first seven days after TECARTUS infusion was 90% (70/78) in patients with ALL.

6. DOSAGE FORMS AND STRENGTHS

TECARTUS is available as a cell suspension for infusion.

• ALL: A single dose of TECARTUS contains 1 x 10^6 CAR-positive viable T cells per kg of body weight [maximum of 1 x 10^8 CAR-positive viable T cells (for patients 100 kg and above)] in approximately 68 mL suspension in an infusion bag.

7. CONTRAINDICATIONS: None

8. WARNINGS AND PRECAUTIONS

5.1. CRS occurred in 92% (72/78) of patients with ALL, including ≥ Grade 3 (Lee grading system1) CRS in 26% of patients. Three patients with ALL had ongoing CRS events at the time of death. The median time to onset of CRS was five days (range 1 to 12 days) and the median duration of CRS was eight days (range 2 to 63 days) for patients with ALL. The incidence of CRS (first occurrence) within the first seven days after TECARTUS infusion was 90% (70/78) in patients with ALL. Ensure that a minimum of two doses of tocilizumab are available for each patient prior to infusion of TECARTUS. Monitor patients daily for at least seven days for patients with MCL and at least 14 days for patients with ALL at the certified healthcare facility following infusion for signs and symptoms of CRS. Monitor patients for signs or symptoms of CRS for four weeks after

9. DOSAGE FORMS AND STRENGTHS

TECARTUS is available as a cell suspension for infusion.

• ALL: A single dose of TECARTUS contains 1 x 10^6 CAR-positive viable T cells per kg of body weight [maximum of 1 x 10^8 CAR-positive viable T cells (for patients 100 kg and above)] in approximately 68 mL suspension in an infusion bag.

10. CONTRAINDICATIONS: None

11. WARNINGS AND PRECAUTIONS

5.1. CRS occurred in 92% (72/78) of patients with ALL, including ≥ Grade 3 (Lee grading system1) CRS in 26% of patients. Three patients with ALL had ongoing CRS events at the time of death. The median time to onset of CRS was five days (range 1 to 12 days) and the median duration of CRS was eight days (range 2 to 63 days) for patients with ALL. The incidence of CRS (first occurrence) within the first seven days after TECARTUS infusion was 90% (70/78) in patients with ALL. Ensure that a minimum of two doses of tocilizumab are available for each patient prior to infusion of TECARTUS. Monitor patients daily for at least 14 days for patients with ALL at the certified healthcare facility following infusion for signs and symptoms of CRS. Monitor patients for signs or symptoms of CRS for four weeks after the infusion.

12. DOSAGE FORMS AND STRENGTHS

TECARTUS is available as a cell suspension for infusion.

• ALL: A single dose of TECARTUS contains 1 x 10^6 CAR-positive viable T cells per kg of body weight [maximum of 1 x 10^8 CAR-positive viable T cells (for patients 100 kg and above)] in approximately 68 mL suspension in an infusion bag.

13. CONTRAINDICATIONS: None

14. WARNINGS AND PRECAUTIONS

Cytokine Release Syndrome (CRS)

CRS occurred in 92% (72/78) of patients with ALL, including ≥ Grade 3 (Lee grading system1) CRS in 26% of patients. Three patients with ALL had ongoing CRS events at the time of death. The median time to onset of CRS was five days (range 1 to 12 days) and the median duration of CRS was eight days (range 2 to 63 days) for patients with ALL. The incidence of CRS (first occurrence) within the first seven days after TECARTUS infusion was 90% (70/78) in patients with ALL. Ensure that a minimum of two doses of tocilizumab are available for each patient prior to infusion of TECARTUS. Monitor patients daily for at least seven days for patients with MCL and at least 14 days for patients with ALL at the certified healthcare facility following infusion for signs and symptoms of CRS. Monitor patients for signs or symptoms of CRS for four weeks after the infusion of TECARTUS.

15. DOSAGE FORMS AND STRENGTHS

TECARTUS is available as a cell suspension for infusion.

• ALL: A single dose of TECARTUS contains 1 x 10^6 CAR-positive viable T cells per kg of body weight [maximum of 1 x 10^8 CAR-positive viable T cells (for patients 100 kg and above)] in approximately 68 mL suspension in an infusion bag.

16. CONTRAINDICATIONS: None

17. WARNINGS AND PRECAUTIONS

Cytokine Release Syndrome (CRS)

CRS occurred in 92% (72/78) of patients with ALL, including ≥ Grade 3 (Lee grading system1) CRS in 26% of patients. Three patients with ALL had ongoing CRS events at the time of death. The median time to onset of CRS was five days (range 1 to 12 days) and the median duration of CRS was eight days (range 2 to 63 days) for patients with ALL. The incidence of CRS (first occurrence) within the first seven days after TECARTUS infusion was 90% (70/78) in patients with ALL. Ensure that a minimum of two doses of tocilizumab are available for each patient prior to infusion of TECARTUS. Monitor patients daily for at least 14 days for patients with ALL at the certified healthcare facility following infusion for signs and symptoms of CRS. Monitor patients for signs or symptoms of CRS for four weeks after infusion. Counsel patients to seek immediate medical attention should signs or symptoms of CRS occur at any time.

18. DOSAGE FORMS AND STRENGTHS

TECARTUS is available as a cell suspension for infusion.

• ALL: A single dose of TECARTUS contains 1 x 10^6 CAR-positive viable T cells per kg of body weight [maximum of 1 x 10^8 CAR-positive viable T cells (for patients 100 kg and above)] in approximately 68 mL suspension in an infusion bag.

19. CONTRAINDICATIONS: None

20. WARNINGS AND PRECAUTIONS

5.1. Cytokine Release Syndrome (CRS) including fatal or life-threatening reactions, occurred following treatment with TECARTUS.

CRS occurred in 92% (72/78) of patients with ALL, including ≥ Grade 3 (Lee grading system1) CRS in 26% of patients. Three patients with ALL had ongoing CRS events at the time of death. The median time to onset of CRS was five days (range 1 to 12 days) and the median duration of CRS was eight days (range 2 to 63 days) for patients with ALL. The incidence of CRS (first occurrence) within the first seven days after TECARTUS infusion was 90% (70/78) in patients with ALL. Ensure that a minimum of two doses of tocilizumab are available for each patient prior to infusion of TECARTUS. Monitor patients daily for at least 14 days for patients with ALL at the certified healthcare facility following infusion for signs and symptoms of CRS. Monitor patients for signs or symptoms of CRS for four weeks after infusion. Counsel patients to seek immediate medical attention should signs or symptoms of CRS occur at any time.

At the first sign of CRS, institute treatment with supportive care, tocilizumab, or tocilizumab and corticosteroids as indicated.

5.2. Neurologic toxicities

Neurologic events, including those that were fatal or life-threatening, occurred following treatment with TECARTUS. Neurologic events occurred in 87% (68/78) of patients with ALL, including ≥ Grade 3 in 35% of patients. The median time to onset for neurologic events was seven days (range 1 to 51 days) with a median duration of 15 days (range 1 to 397 days) in patients with ALL. Five (6%) patients did not experience CRS with neurologic events and eight patients (10%) developed neurological events after the resolution of CRS. Neurologic events resolved for 119 out of 134 (89%) patients treated with TECARTUS. Six patients with ALL had ongoing neurologic events at the time of death. For patients with ALL, neurologic events occurred before, during, and after CRS in 4 (5%), 57 (73%), and 8 (10%) of patients, respectively. Three patients (4%) had neurologic events without CRS. The onset of neurologic events can be concurrent with CRS, following resolution of CRS or in the absence of CRS. The incidence of neurologic events (first occurrence) within the first seven days after TECARTUS infusion was 55% (43/78) in patients with ALL. Monitor patients daily for at least seven days for patients with MCL and at least 14 days for patients with ALL at the certified healthcare facility following infusion for signs and symptoms of neurologic toxicities. Monitor patients for signs or symptoms of neurologic toxicities for four weeks after infusion and treat promptly.

5.3. **YESCARTA and TECARTUS REMS Program**

Because of the risk of CRS and neurologic toxicities, TECARTUS is available only through a restricted program under a Risk Evaluation and Mitigation Strategy (REMS) called the YESCARTA and TECARTUS REMS Program.

The required components of the YESCARTA and TECARTUS REMS Program are

• Healthcare facilities that dispense and administer TECARTUS must be enrolled and comply with the REMS requirements. Certified healthcare facilities must have on-site, immediate access to tocilizumab, and ensure that a minimum of two doses of tocilizumab are available for each patient for infusion within two hours after TECARTUS infusion, if needed for treatment of CRS.

• Certified healthcare facilities must ensure that healthcare providers who prescribe, dispense, or administer TECARTUS are trained in the management of CRS and neurologic toxicities. Further information is available at www.YescartaTecartus REMS.com or 1-844-454-KITE (5483).

5.4. Hemophagocytic lymphohistiocytosis/macrophage activation syndrome

Hemophagocytic lymphohistiocytosis/macrophage activation syndrome (HLH/MAS) including life-threatening reactions, occurred following treatment with TECARTUS. HLH/MAS occurred in 4% (3/78) of patients with ALL. Two patients experienced Grade 3 events and 1 patient experienced a Grade 4 event. The median time to onset for HLH/MAS was 8 days (range: 6 to 9 days) with a median duration of 5 days (range: 2 to 8 days). All three patients with HLH/MAS had concurrent CRS symptoms and neurologic events after TECARTUS infusion. Treatment of HLH/MAS should be administered per institutional standards.

*[Author's note: the information below on HLH and MAS is **NOT** in the FDA label for Tecartus. It is inserted here to give further clinical details on HLH and MAS]*

*[**Hemophagocytic lymphohistiocytosis** (HLH), also known as haemophagocytic lymphohistiocytosis (British spelling), and hemophagocytic or haemophagocytic syndrome, is an uncommon hematologic disorder seen more often in children than in adults. It is a life-threatening disease of severe hyperinflammation caused by uncontrolled proliferation of activated lymphocytes and macrophages, characterised by proliferation of morphologically benign lymphocytes and macrophages that secrete high amounts of inflammatory cytokines. It is classified as ono of the **cytokine storm syndromes.** There are inherited and non-inherited (acquired) causes of hemophagocytic lymphohistiocytosis. The onset of HLH occurs before the age of one year in approximately 70 percent of cases. Familial HLH should be suspected if siblings are diagnosed with HLH or if symptoms recur when therapy has been stopped. Familial HLH is an autosomal recessive disease, hence each sibling of a child with familial HLH has a twenty-five–percent chance of developing the disease, a fifty-percent chance of carrying the defective gene (which is very rarely associated with any risk of disease), and a twenty-five–percent chance of not being affected and not carrying the gene defect.*

Patients with HLH, especially when untreated, may need intensive therapy. Therefore, HLH should be included in the differential diagnosis of intensive care unit patients with cytopenia and hyperferritinemia. Patients in the earlier stages of HLH are frequently hospitalized at internal medicine wards.

HLH clinically manifests with fever, enlargement of the liver and spleen, enlarged lymph nodes, yellow discoloration of the skin and eyes, and a rash. Laboratory findings may include elevated triglyceride levels, low fibrinogen levels, transaminitis, and elevated ferritin levels (among others)

The underlying cause oh HLH leads to an unchecked immune response. Impaired NK-cell cytotoxicity is the hallmark of HLH. All genetic defects for familial HLH are related to granule-dependent cytotoxicity. This inability to remove infected and antigen-presenting cells and terminate the immune response leads to uncontrolled proliferation and activation of the immune system with release of excessive cytokines. These cells then infiltrate organs, releasing more cytokines, which gives the clinical picture. The fever is caused by the pro-inflammatory cytokines IL-1, IL-6 and TNF-alpha; the cytopenia is due to the suppressive effect on hematopoiesis by TNF-alpha and TNF-gamma. TNF-alpha and TNF-gamma may also lead to inhibition of lipoprotein lipase or stimulate triglyceride synthesis. Activated macrophages secrete ferritin and plasminogen activator leading to hyperfibrinolysis.

The blood count typically shows decreased numbers of blood cells - including a decreased number of circulating red blood cells, white blood cells, and platelets. The bone marrow may show hemophagocytosis. The liver function tests are usually elevated. A low level of the protein albumin in the blood is common.

The serum C reactive protein, erythrocyte sedimentation rate, and ferritin level are markedly elevated. In children, a ferritin above 10000 is very sensitive and specific for the diagnosis of HLH, however, the diagnostic utility for ferritin is less for adult HLH patients. The serum fibrinogen level is usually low and the D-dimer level is elevated. The sphingomyelinase is elevated.

Diagnostic criteria for acquired HLH are

Fulfillment of five out of the eight criteria below:

Fever (defined as a temperature >100.3 °F, >38 °C)

Enlargement of the spleen

Decreased blood cell counts affecting at least two of three lineages in the peripheral blood:

Haemoglobin <9 g/100 ml (in infants <4 weeks: haemoglobin <10 g/100 ml) (anemia)

Platelets <100×10^9/L (thrombocytopenia)

Neutrophils <1×10^9/L (neutropenia)

High blood levels of triglycerides (fasting, greater than or equal to 265 mg/100 ml) and/or decreased amounts of fibrinogen in the blood (≤ 150 mg/100 ml)

Ferritin ≥ 500 ng/ml

Haemophagocytosis in the bone marrow, spleen or lymph nodes

Low or absent natural killer cell activity

Soluble CD25 (Figure 62), (soluble IL-2 receptor) >2400 U/ml (or per local reference laboratory)

In addition, in the case of familial HLH, no evidence of malignancy should be apparent. Not all five out of eight criteria are required for diagnosis of HLH in adults, and a high index of suspicion is required for diagnosis as delay results in increased mortality. The diagnostic criteria were developed in pediatric populations and have not been validated for adult HLH patients. Attempts to improve diagnosis of HLH have included use of the HScore, which can be used to estimate an individual's risk of HLH. In adults, soluble IL-2 receptor has been found to be a very sensitive marker for HLH, demonstrating 100%

sensitivity for ruling out HLH below a cutoff of 2400 U/mL and optimal cutoff for ruling in at 2515 U/mL (sensitivity, 100%; specificity, 72.5%), with 93% specificity at >10 000 U/mL.

The first case report of HLH was published in 1952 by James Farquar and colleagues].

*[**Macrophage activation syndrome***

*Macrophage activation syndrome is a severe, potentially life-threatening, complication of several chronic rheumatic diseases of childhood. It occurs most commonly with systemic-onset juvenile idiopathic arthritis (SoJIA). In addition, MAS has been described in association with systemic lupus erythematosus (SLE), Kawasaki disease, and adult-onset Still's disease. **It is thought to be closely related and pathophysiologically very similar to reactive (secondary) hemophagocytic lymphohistiocytosis (HLH)** The incidence of MAS is unknown as there is a wide spectrum of clinical manifestations, and episodes may remain unrecognized. The hallmark clinical and laboratory features include high fever, hepatosplenomegaly, lymphadenopathy, pancytopenia, liver dysfunction, **disseminated intravascular coagulation**, hypofibrinogenemia, hyperferritinemia, and hypertriglyceridemia. Despite marked systemic inflammation, the erythrocyte sedimentation rate (ESR) is paradoxically depressed, caused by low fibrinogen levels. The low ESR helps to distinguish the disorder from a flare of the underlying rheumatic disorder, in which case the ESR is usually elevated. A bone marrow biopsy or aspirate usually shows hemophagocytosis. In many cases a trigger is identified, often a viral infection, or a **medication**. There is uncontrolled activation and proliferation of macrophages, and T lymphocytes, with a marked increase in circulating cytokines, such as IFN-gamma, and GM-CSF. The underlying causative event is unclear, and is the subject of ongoing research. In many cases of MAS, a decreased natural killer cell (NK-cell) function is found.*

Disseminated intravascular coagulation: disseminated intravascular coagulation (DIC) is a condition in which blood clots form throughout the body, blocking small blood vessels. Symptoms may include chest pain, shortness of breath, leg pain, problems speaking, or problems moving parts of the body. As clotting factors and platelets are used up, bleeding may occur. This may include blood in the urine, blood in the stool, or bleeding into the skin. Complications may include organ failure.

A febrile patient with known or suspected sJia must be considered for macrophage activation if:

Ferritin >684 ng/ml

and any 2 of the following:

Hemoglobin <90g/L (in infants <4 weeks: <100g/L)

Platelets <100 x 10^9/L

Neutrophils <1.0 x 10^9/L

Fasting triglycerides ≥3.0 mmol/L (i.e., ≥ 265 mg/dl)

Fibrinogen ≤1.5 g/L[3]

The peripheral blood smear may show fragmented red blood cells (known as schistocytes (Figure 63)) due to shear stress from thrombi. However, this finding is neither sensitive nor specific for DIC

In addition, other specific markers of macrophage activation (e.g. soluble CD163), and lymphocyte activation (e.g. soluble IL-2 receptor) can be helpful. NK cell function analysis may show depressed NK function, or, flow cytometry may show a depressed NK cell population.CD163 is the high affinity scavenger receptor for the hemoglobin-haptoglobin complex (Figure 64)

The best treatment for MAS has not been firmly established. Most commonly used treatments include high-dose glucocorticoids, and cyclosporine. In refractory cases treatment regimens are used similar to that in HLH. Anakinra may also be effective].

b. Hypersensitivity reactions

Serious hypersensitivity reactions, including anaphylaxis, may occur due to dimethyl sulfoxide (DMSO) or residual gentamicin in TECARTUS.

Severe infections

Severe or life-threatening infections occurred in patients after TECARTUS infusion. Infections (all grades) occurred in 44% (34/78) of patients with ALL. Grade 3 or higher infections, including bacterial, viral, and fungal infections, occurred in 30% of patients with ALL. TECARTUS should not be administered to patients with clinically significant active systemic infections. Monitor patients for signs and symptoms of infection before and after TECARTUS infusion and treat appropriately. Administer prophylactic antimicrobials according to local guidelines. Febrile neutropenia was observed in 35% of patients with ALL after TECARTUS infusion and may be concurrent with CRS. The febrile neutropenia in 27 (35%) of patients with ALL includes events of “febrile neutropenia” (11 (14%)) plus the concurrent events of “fever” and “neutropenia” (16 (21%)). In the event of febrile neutropenia, evaluate for infection and manage with broad spectrum antibiotics, fluids, and other supportive care as medically indicated. In immunosuppressed patients, life-threatening and fatal opportunistic infections have been reported. The possibility of rare infectious etiologies (e.g., fungal and viral infections such as HHV-6 and progressive multifocal leukoencephalopathy) should be considered in patients with neurologic events and appropriate diagnostic evaluations should be performed.

Hepatitis B reactivation

Hepatitis B virus (HBV) reactivation, in some cases resulting in fulminant hepatitis, hepatic failure, and death, can occur in patients treated with drugs directed against B cells. Perform screening for HBV, hepatitis C virus (HCV), and human immunodeficiency virus (HIV) in accordance with clinical guidelines before collection of cells for manufacturing.

[Author's note: this information is NOT in the FDA label for TECARTUS.

[Figure 16. Hepatitis B viral antigens and antibodies detectable in the blood following acute infection

This image is by User:GrahamColm - Own work, Public Domain, https://commons.wikimedia.org/w/index.php?curid=23165261; https://en.wikipedia.org/wiki/Hepatitis_B#/media/File:HBV_serum_markers.png. This work has been released into the public domain by its author, GrahamColm. No changes were made to this image.

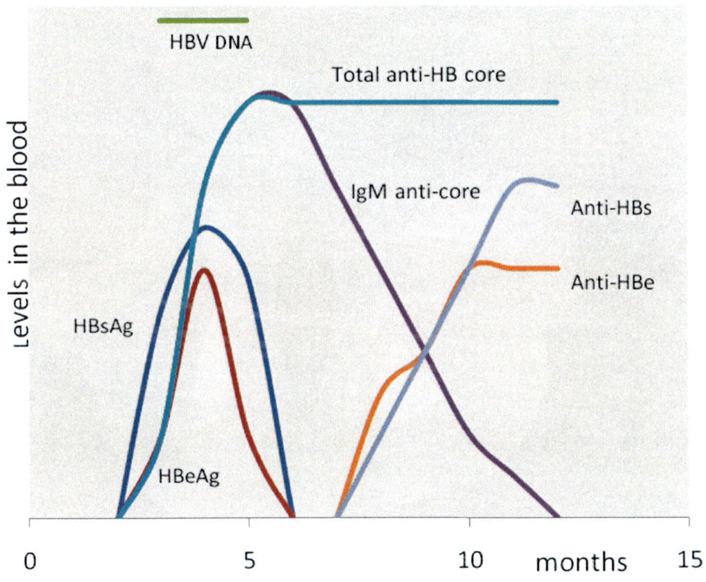

5.7. Prolonged cytopenias

Patients may exhibit cytopenias for several weeks following lymphodepleting chemotherapy and TECARTUS infusion. In patients with ALL who were responders to TECARTUS treatment, Grade 3 or higher cytopenias not resolved by Day 30 following TECARTUS infusion occurred in 20% (7/35) of the patients and included neutropenia (12%) and thrombocytopenia (12%); Grade 3 or higher cytopenias not resolved by Day 60 following TECARTUS infusion occurred in 11% (4/35) of the patients and included neutropenia (9%) and thrombocytopenia (6%). Monitor blood counts after TECARTUS infusion.

5.8. Hypogammaglobulinemia

B cell aplasia and hypogammaglobulinemia can occur in patients receiving treatment with TECARTUS. Hypogammaglobulinemia was reported in 9% (7/78) of patients with ALL. Monitor immunoglobulin levels after treatment with TECARTUS and manage using infection precautions, antibiotic prophylaxis, and immunoglobulin replacement. The safety of immunization with live viral vaccines during or following TECARTUS treatment has not been studied. Vaccination with live virus vaccines is not recommended for at least six weeks prior to the start of lymphodepleting chemotherapy, during TECARTUS treatment, and until immune recovery following treatment with TECARTUS.

5.9. Secondary malignancies

Patients treated with TECARTUS may develop secondary malignancies. Monitor life-long for secondary malignancies. In the event that a secondary malignancy occurs, contact Kite at 1-844-454-KITE (5483) to obtain instructions on patient samples to collect for testing.

5.10. Effects on ability to drive and use machines

Due to the potential for neurologic events, including altered mental status or seizures, patients receiving TECARTUS are at risk for altered or decreased consciousness or coordination in the eight weeks following TECARTUS infusion. Advise patients to refrain from driving and engaging in hazardous occupations or activities, such as operating heavy or potentially dangerous machinery, during this initial period.

6. ADVERSE REACTIONS

The following clinically significant adverse reactions are described elsewhere in the labeling:

- Cytokine Release Syndrome [see Warnings and Precautions (5.1)]

- Neurologic Toxicities [see Warnings and Precautions (5.2)]
- Hemophagocytic Lymphohistiocytosis/Macrophage Activation Syndrome [see Warnings and Precautions (5.4)]
- Hypersensitivity Reactions [see Warnings and Precautions (5.5)]
- Severe Infections [see Warnings and Precautions (5.6)]
- Prolonged Cytopenias [see Warnings and Precautions (5.7)]
- Hypogammaglobulinemia [see Warnings and Precautions (5.8)]

6.2. Clinical trials experience

Because clinical trials are conducted under widely varying conditions, adverse reaction rates observed in the clinical trials of a drug cannot be directly compared to rates in the clinical trials of another drug and may not reflect the rates observed in practice.

Patients with Relapsed/Refractory B-cell precursor Acute Lymphoblastic Leukemia (ALL)

The safety of TECARTUS was evaluated in a Phase 1/2 open-label, multicenter study (ZUMA-3) in which a total of 78 patients with relapsed/refractory ALL received a single dose of CAR-positive T cells (1×10^6 anti- CD19 CAR T cells/kg) that was weight-based [see Clinical Studies (14.2)].

The most common non-laboratory adverse reactions (≥ 20%) were fever, cytokine release syndrome, hypotension, encephalopathy, tachycardia, nausea, chills, headache, fatigue, febrile neutropenia, diarrhea, musculoskeletal pain, hypoxia, rash, edema, tremor, infection with pathogen unspecified, constipation, decreased appetite, and vomiting. The most common serious adverse reactions (≥ 2%) were cytokine release syndrome, febrile neutropenia, hypotension, encephalopathy, fever, infection with pathogen unspecified, hypoxia, tachycardia, bacterial infections, respiratory failure, seizure, diarrhea, dyspnea, fungal infections, viral infections, coagulopathy, delirium, fatigue, hemophagocytic lymphohistiocytosis, musculoskeletal pain, edema, and paraparesis.

The most common (≥ 10%) Grade 3 or 4 reactions were fever, febrile neutropenia, hypotension, encephalopathy, cytokine release syndrome, hypoxia, and infection with pathogen unspecified. Fatal adverse reactions occurred in 5% (4/78) of patients including cerebral edema, sepsis, and fungal pneumonia. Of the 4 patients who had fatal adverse reactions: one patient with fatal pneumonia had pre-existing pneumonia prior to study enrollment, and one patient with fatal sepsis had prolonged cytopenia and immunosuppression from prior therapies and underlying disease.

Table 5 summarizes the adverse reactions (excluding laboratory abnormalities) that occurred in at least 10% of patients treated with TECARTUS and Table 6 describes the laboratory abnormalities of Grade 3 or 4 that occurred in at least 10% of patients.

Table 5. Summary of Adverse Reactions Observed in at Least 10% of Patients Treated with TECARTUS in ZUMA-3 (N=78)

Adverse Reaction	Any Grade (%)	Grade 3 or Higher (%)
Blood and Lymphatic System Disorders		
Febrile Neutropenia[a]	35	35
Coagulopathy[b]	17	5
Cardiac Disorders		
Tachycardias[c]	63	6
Arrhythmia[d]	15	1
Gastrointestinal Disorders		
Nausea	41	1
Diarrhea	32	6
Abdominal pain[e]	19	0
Constipation	24	0
Vomiting	21	3
General Disorders and Administration Site Conditions		
Fever	96	38
Chills	40	0
Edema[f]	29	5
Fatigue[g]	37	1
Pain	13	1

Immune System Disorders		
Cytokine release syndrome	92	26
Infections and Infestations		
Infection with pathogen unspecified[h]	28	22
Bacterial infections[i]	15	8
Fungal infections[j]	13	5
Metabolism and Nutrition Disorders		
Decreased appetite	22	1
Musculoskeletal and Connective Tissue Disorders		
Musculoskeletal pain[k]	32	5
Muscular weakness	14	1
Nervous System Disorders		
Encephalopathy[l]	63	27
Headache	38	1
Tremor	29	1
Dizziness[m]	13	1
Psychiatric Disorders		
Delirium[n]	18	5
Anxiety	12	0
Insomnia	13	0
Respiratory, Thoracic and Mediastinal Disorders		
Hypoxia	31	23
Cough[o]	12	0

Dyspnea	12	1

Adverse Reaction	Any Grade (%)	Grade 3 or Higher (%)
Skin and Subcutaneous Tissue Disorders		
Rash[p]	31	0
Vascular Disorders		
Hypotension[q]	69	33
Hemorrhage[r]	13	4
Hypertension	13	6

[a]Febrile neutropenia includes febrile neutropenia (11 (14%)) and fever occurring concurrently with neutropenia events (16 (21%)).

[b]Coagulopathy includes blood fibrinogen decreased, coagulopathy, disseminated intravascular coagulation, hypofibrinogenemia, international normalized ratio increased.

[c]Tachycardias includes sinus tachycardia, tachycardia.

[d]Arrhythmia includes arrhythmia, arrhythmia supraventricular, atrial fibrillation, atrial flutter, atrial tachycardia,bradycardia, cardiac arrest, electrocardiogram QT prolonged, electrocardiogram T wave inversion, pulseless electrical activity, sinus bradycardia, supraventricular tachycardia, ventricular tachycardia.

[e]Abdominal pain includes abdominal discomfort, abdominal pain, abdominal pain upper.

[f]Edema includes face edema, fluid overload, generalized edema, edema, edema peripheral, swelling face, tongue edema.

[g]Fatigue includes asthenia, cancer fatigue, fatigue, malaise.

[h]Infection with pathogen unspecified includes, catheter bacteremia, conjunctivitis, device related infection, mucosal infection, nasopharyngitis, parotitis, pneumonia, sepsis, septic shock, sinusitis, upper respiratory tract infection, urinary tract infection.

[i]Bacterial infections includes bacteremia, bacterial disease carrier, cellulitis, cellulitis of male external genital organ, clostridial infection, clostridium difficile colitis, clostridium difficile infection, enterococcal

bacteremia, enterococcal infection, escherichia bacteremia, escherichia infection, escherichia sepsis, pseudomonas infection, staphylococcal bacteremia, staphylococcal infection, wound infection staphylococcal.

[j]Fungal infections includes bronchopulmonary aspergillosis, candida infection, fungal skin infection, mycotic oral candidiasis, osteomyelitis fungal, pneumocystis jirovecii pneumonia, pneumonia fungal, sinusitis fungal.

[k]Musculoskeletal pain includes arthralgia, back pain, bone pain, coccydynia, muscle strain, musculoskeletal chest pain, musculoskeletal pain, myalgia, neck pain, non-cardiac chest pain, pain in extremity.

[l]Encephalopathy includes altered state of consciousness, aphasia, cognitive disorder, confusional state, depressed level of consciousness, disturbance in attention, dysarthria, dysgraphia, encephalopathy, immune effector cell -associated neurotoxicity syndrome, memory impairment, mental status changes, slow response to stimuli, slow speech, somnolence, speech disorder.

[m]Dizziness includes dizziness, syncope.

[n]Delirium includes agitation, delirium, delusion, disorientation, hallucination.

[o]Cough includes cough, productive cough.

[p]Rash includes catheter site urticaria, dermatitis bullous, drug eruption, pruritus, rash, rash macular, rash maculo-papular, rash pustular, toxic skin eruption, urticaria.

[q]Hypotension includes hypotension, orthostatic hypotension.

[r]Hemorrhage includes conjunctival hemorrhage, contusion, epistaxis, gastric hemorrhage,hematoma, hematoma muscle, hemorrhage intracranial, hemorrhoidal hemorrhage, menorrhagia, petechiae, pulmonary alveolar hemorrhage, retinal hemorrhage, vaginal hemorrhage, vitreous hemorrhage

Other clinically important adverse reactions that occurred in less than 10% of patients treated with TECARTUS include the following:

Cardiac disorder: cardiac failure (4%), palpitations (3%)

Eye disorders: visual impairment (9%)

Gastrointestinal disorders: dry mouth (6%), dysphagia (4%), oral pain (1%)

Immune system disorders: hypogammaglobulinemia (9%), hemophagocytic lymphohistiocytosis (4%), drug hypersensitivity (1%)

Infections and infestations: viral infections (6%)

Metabolism and nutrition disorders: dehydration (5%), tumor lysis syndrome (1%)

Musculoskeletal and connective tissue disorders: muscle spasms (4%), musculoskeletal stiffness (3%)

Nervous system disorders: seizure (8%), ataxia (5%), peripheral neuropathy (4%), myoclonus (3%), paraparesis (3%), brain edema (1%), brain herniation (1%), cauda equina syndrome (1%),

monoplegia (1%)

Renal and urinary disorders: renal impairment (6%)

Respiratory, thoracic and mediastinal disorders: respiratory failure (9%), pulmonary edema (6%), pleural effusion (4%), pneumonitis (4%)

Skin and subcutaneous tissue disorders: skin lesion (4%), decubitus ulcer (3%), dry skin (3%), skin ulcer (3%), alopecia (1%), hyperhidrosis (1%), skin hyperpigmentation (1%)

Vascular disorders: thrombosis (4%)

Table 6. Grade 3 or 4 Laboratory Abnormalities Occurring in ≥ 10% of Patients in ZUMA-3 Following TECARTUS Infusion (N = 78)

Grades 3 or 4 (%)	
Leukopenia	99
Neutropenia	97
Lymphopenia	96
Thrombocytopenia	87
Anemia	77
Hypophosphatemia	47
Alanine aminotransferase increased	31

Aspartate aminotransferase increased	23
Hyperglycemia	22
Hypocalcemia	22
Blood uric acid increased	19
Direct bilirubin increased	19
Hyponatremia	19
Hypokalemia	13
Hyperbilirubinemia	10

6.2. Immunogenicity

TECARTUS has the potential to induce anti-product antibodies, which has been evaluated using an enzyme-linked immunosorbent assay (ELISA) for the detection of binding antibodies against FMC63, the originating antibody of the anti-CD19 CAR. Based on an initial screening assay in ZUMA-3, 16 of 100 patients tested positive for antibodies at any time point. Among patients with evaluable samples for confirmatory testing, two patients were confirmed to be antibody-positive after treatment. One of the two patients had a confirmed positive antibody result at Month 6. The second patient had a confirmed antibody result at retreatment Day 28 and Month 3. There is no evidence that the kinetics of initial expansion and persistence of TECARTUS, or the safety or effectiveness of TECARTUS, were altered in these patients.

8. USE IN SPECIFIC POPULATIONS

8.1. Pregnancy

Risk summary

There are no available data with TECARTUS use in pregnant women. No animal reproductive and developmental toxicity studies have been conducted with TECARTUS to assess whether TECARTUS can cause fetal harm when administered to a pregnant woman. It is not known if TECARTUS has the potential to be transferred to the fetus. Based on the mechanism of action of TECARTUS, if the transduced cells cross the placenta, they may cause fetal toxicity, including B cell lymphocytopenia. Therefore, TECARTUS is not recommended for women who are pregnant. Pregnancy after TECARTUS infusion should be discussed with the treating physician. In the U.S. general population, the estimated background risk of major birth defects and miscarriage in clinically recognized pregnancies is 2% - 4% and 15% - 20%, respectively.

8.2. Lactation

Risk summary

There is no information regarding the presence of TECARTUS in human milk, the effect on the breastfed infant, and the effects on milk production. The developmental and health benefits of breastfeeding should be considered along with the mother's clinical need for TECARTUS and any potential adverse effects on the breastfed infant from TECARTUS or from the underlying maternal condition.

8.3. Females and males of reproductive potential

Pregnancy testing

Pregnancy status of females with reproductive potential should be verified. Sexually active females of reproductive potential should have a negative pregnancy test prior to starting treatment with TECARTUS.

Contraception

See the Prescribing Information for fludarabine and cyclophosphamide for information on the need for effective contraception in patients who receive the lymphodepleting chemotherapy. There are insufficient exposure data to provide a recommendation concerning duration of contraception following treatment with TECARTUS.

Infertility

There are no data on the effect of TECARTUS on fertility.

8.4. Pediatric use

The safety and efficacy of TECARTUS have not been established in pediatric patients.

8.5. Geriatric use

Of the 78 patients treated with TECARTUS for ALL, 12 (15%) were 65 years of age and over. No overall differences in safety or effectiveness were observed between these patients and younger patients.

11. DESCRIPTION

TECARTUS (brexucabtagene autoleucel) is a CD19-directed genetically modified autologous T cell immunotherapy. To prepare TECARTUS, a patient's own T cells are harvested and genetically modified ex vivo by retroviral transduction to express a chimeric antigen receptor (CAR) comprising a murine anti-CD19 single-chain variable fragment (scFv) linked to CD28 and CD3-zeta co-stimulatory domains. The anti-CD19 CAR T cells are expanded and infused back into the patient, where they can recognize and eliminate CD19- expressing target cells.

TECARTUS is prepared from the patient's peripheral blood mononuclear cells, which are obtained via a standard leukapheresis procedure. The mononuclear cells are enriched for T cells and activated with anti-CD3 and anti-CD28 antibodies in the presence of IL-2, then transduced with a replication-incompetent retroviral vector containing the anti-CD19 CAR transgene. The transduced T cells are expanded in cell culture, washed, formulated into a suspension, and cryopreserved. The manufacture of TECARTUS includes a T cell enrichment step that may reduce the likelihood of circulating CD19-expressing tumor cells in patients' leukapheresis material driving the activation, expansion, and exhaustion of the anti-CD19 CAR T cells during the ex vivo manufacturing process. The product must pass a sterility test before release for shipping as a frozen suspension in a patient-specific infusion bag. The product is thawed prior to infusion [see Dosage and Administration (2.2),

How Supplied/Storage and Handling

In addition to T cells, TECARTUS may contain natural killer (NK) cells. The formulation contains CryoStor (dimethyl sulfoxide [DMSO], final concentration, 5%), sodium chloride (NaCl), and Human Serum Albumin (HSA).

12. CLINICAL PHARMACOLOGY

12.1. Mechanism of Action

TECARTUS, a CD19-directed genetically modified autologous T cell immunotherapy, binds to CD19-expressing cancer cells and normal B cells. Studies demonstrated that following anti-CD19 CAR T cell engagement with CD19-expressing target cells, the CD28 and CD3-zeta co-stimulatory domains activate downstream signaling cascades that lead to T cell activation, proliferation, acquisition of effector functions, and secretion of inflammatory cytokines and chemokines. This sequence of events leads to killing of CD19- expressing cells.

12.2. Pharmacodynamics

After TECARTUS infusion, pharmacodynamic responses were evaluated over a four-week interval by measuring transient elevation of cytokines, chemokines, and other molecules in blood. Levels of cytokines and chemokines such as IL-6, IL-8, IL-10, IL-15, TNF-α, IFN-γ, and sIL2Rα were analyzed. Peak elevation was generally observed within 8 days after infusion, and levels generally returned to baseline within 28 days.

Due to the on-target effect of TECARTUS, a period of B cell aplasia is expected.

12.3. Pharmacokinetics

Following infusion (target dose of 1 x 106 anti-CD19 CAR T cells/kg) of TECARTUS in ZUMA-3 (Phase 2), anti-CD19 CAR T cells exhibited an initial rapid expansion followed by a decline to near baseline levels by 6 months. Median anti- CD19 CAR T-cell time to peak was 15 days after TECARTUS infusion.

Description of Pharmacokinetics in Adult r/r B-cell precursor ALL

Median peak anti-CD19 CAR T-cell levels over time by best overall response per independent review was 38.4 cells/μL (range: 1.31 to 1,533.4 cells/μL; n = 32) in patients who had overall complete remission (CR+CRi), and 0.5 cells/μL (range: 0.00 to 183.5 cells/μL, n = 17) in patients who had non-complete remission. The median AUC 0-28 in patients who had overall complete remission (CR+CRi) was 424.0 cells/μL•days (range: 14.12 to 19,390.4 cells/μL

•days; n = 32) vs 7.9 cells/μL•days in patients who had non-complete remission (range: 0.00 to 889.0 cells/μL•days; n=17).

Median peak anti-CD19 CAR T-cell and AUC 0-28 levels in patients who received neither corticosteroids nor tocilizumab (peak 5.7 cells/μL; AUC 0-28: 60.7 cells/μL•days, n=11) were higher than patients who received corticosteroids alone (peak: 36.2 cells/ μL; AUC_{0-28}: 423.1 cells/μL•days, n= 1); both groups were lower than evaluable patients who received tocilizumab alone (peak 11.2 cells/ μL; AUC_{0-28}: 137.4 cells/μL•days, n=9); the highest exposure was in evaluable patients who received both corticosteroids and tocilizumab (peak: 49.2 cells/μL; AUC $_{0-28}$: 454.1 cells/ μL•days, n=34).

Hepatic and renal impairment studies of TECARTUS were not conducted.

13. NONCLINICAL TOXICOLOGY

13.1. Carcinogenesis, Mutagenesis, Impairment of Fertility

No carcinogenicity or genotoxicity studies have been conducted with TECARTUS. No studies have been conducted to evaluate the effects of TECARTUS on fertility.

14. CLINICAL STUDIES

14.1. Relapsed or Refractory B-cell precursor Acute Lymphoblastic Leukemia

The efficacy of TECARTUS was evaluated in ZUMA-3 (NCT02614066), an open-label, single-arm, multicenter trial in adult patients with relapsed or refractory B-cell precursor acute lymphoblastic leukemia (ALL). Eligible patients were adults with primary refractory ALL, first relapse following a remission lasting ≤ 12 months, relapsed or refractory ALL after second-line or higher therapy, or relapsed or refractory ALL at least 100 days after allogeneic stem cell transplantation (HSCT). The study excluded patients with active or serious infections, active graft-vs-host disease or taking immunosuppressive medications within 4 weeks prior to enrollment, and any history of CNS disorders, including CNS-2 disease with neurologic changes and CNS-3 disease irrespective of neurological changes. Treatment consisted of lymphodepleting chemotherapy (fludarabine 25 mg/m^2 iv daily on Days -4, -3 and -2; cyclophosphamide 900 mg/m^2 iv on Day -2) followed by a single intravenous infusion of TECARTUS at a target dose of 1×10^6 anti-CD19 CAR T cells/kg (maximum 1×10^8 cells) on Day 0. All treated patients were hospitalized until at least Day 7. Seventy-one patients were enrolled and leukapheresed; six of these patients did not receive TECARTUS due to manufacturing failure, eight patients were not treated primarily due to adverse events following leukapheresis, two patients underwent leukapheresis and received lymphodepleting chemotherapy but were not treated with TECARTUS, and one patient treated with TECARTUS was inevaluable for efficacy. Among the remaining 54 efficacy-evaluable patients, the median time from leukapheresis to product delivery was 16 days (range: 11 to 39 days) and the median time from leukapheresis to TECARTUS infusion was 29 days (range: 20 to 60 days). Of the 54 patients who were efficacy evaluable, the median age was 40 years (range: 19 to 84 years), 61% were male, and 67% were White, 6% were Asian, 2% were Black or African American, and 2% were American Indian or Alaska Native. At enrollment, 46% had refractory relapse, 26% had primary refractory disease, 20% had untreated second or later relapse, and 7% had first untreated relapse. Among prior therapies, 43% of patients were previously treated with allo-HSCT, 46% with blinatumomab, and 22% with inotuzumab. Twenty-six percent of patients were Philadelphia chromosome positive (Ph+). Fifty (93%) patients had received bridging therapy between leukapheresis and lymphodepleting chemotherapy to control disease burden. The efficacy of TECARTUS was established on the basis of complete remission (CR) within 3 months after infusion and the duration of CR (DOCR). Twenty-eight (51.9%) of the 54 evaluable patients achieved CR, and with a median follow-up for responders of 7.1 months, the median DOCR was not reached (Table 8). The median time to CR was 56 days (range: 25 to 86 days). All efficacy evaluable patients had potential follow-up for ≥ 10 months with a median actual follow-up time of 12.3 months (range: 0.3 to 22.1 months).

Table 8: Efficacy Results in Adult Patients with Relapsed/Refractory B-cell precursor ALL

	Efficacy Evaluable Patients[a] **N= 54**	**All Leukapheresed Patients** **N = 71**
OCR rate (CR + CRi), n (%) [95% CI]	35 (64.8) [51, 77]	36 (50.7) [39, 63]
CR rate, n (%) [95% CI]	28 (51.9) [37.8, 65.7]	29 (40.9) [29.3, 53.2]
Duration of Remission, Median in months [95% CI] (Range[b] in months)	13.6 [9.4, NE] (0.03+, 16.07+)	13.6 [8.7, NE] (0.03+, 16.07+)
DOR, if best response is CR, median in months [95% CI] (Range in months)	NR [9.6, NE] (0.03+, 16.07+)	13.6 [9.4, NE] (0.03+, 16.07+)
DOR, if best response is CRi, median in months [95% CI] (Range in months)	8.7 [1.0, NE] (0.03+, 10.15+)	8.7 [1.0, NE] (0.03+, 10.15+)
Median Follow-up for CR in months	7.1 (0.03+, 16.1+)	5.0 (0.03+, 16.1+)

[a]Of the 71 patients that were enrolled (and leukapheresed), 57 patients received lymphodepleting chemotherapy, and 55 patients received TECARTUS. 54 patients were included in the efficacy evaluable population.

[b]A + sign indicates a censored value.

Abbreviations used: CI, confidence interval; CR, complete remission; CRi, complete remission with incomplete blood count recovery; DOR, duration of remission; NE, not estimable; NR, not reached, OCR, overall complete remission; NE, not estimable

15. Allogeneic CAR T cells

Since currently available CAR T cells are made from the patient's own (autologous) T cells – personalized therapy – their manufacturing is very expensive with courses costing hundreds of thousand of US dollars. One way to reduce cost is to make CAR T cells from normal volunteer donors, where 1 production run should provide enough CAR T cells for a number of recipients. Progress is already being made in this are with two additional gene engineering of the cells: firstly, using a base-editing tool such as CRISPER (clustered regulatory interspaced short palindromic repeats)/Cas9.

By delivering the Cas9 nuclease complexed with a synthetic guide RNA (gRNA) into a cell, the cell's genome can be cut at a desired location, allowing existing genes to be removed and/or new ones added in vivo without risk of causing unwanted mutations. Genes targeted by CRISPR or similar technologies, such as simultaneous transcription activator-like effector nuclease (TALEN), allow gene editing of the T cell receptor α chain (to minimize the risk of GVHD), β2microglobulin (to minimize the risk of rejection of the infused allogeneic CAR T cells and CD52 gene loci to effect lymphodepletion. Such cells have already been used successfully in two infants with refractory ALL before high dose conditioning prior to a successful allogeneic hematopoietic stem cell transplantation. This bridge-to-transplantation strategy demonstrated the therapeutic potential of gene-editing technology.

16. CONCLUSIONS

The first cellular therapy that entered mainstream medicine was hematopoietic stem cell transplantation in the 1970s. Other cell types have been tried such as natural killer cells, neutrophils and mesenchymal cells but none are in standard practice with the possible exception of neutrophils in people with febrile neutropenia or severe infection due to neutropenia who are unresponsive to antimicrobial agents plus granulocyte colony-stimulating factor (G-CSF).

CAR T cells are generating intense interest with hematologists and oncologists because of their remarkable ability to induce significant responses in people with acute B cell leukemia, as well as diffuse large B cell lymphoma, mantle cell lymphoma and multiple myeloma refractory or resistant to currently available treatment including drugs, irradiation, monoclonal antibodies and, in some cases, hematopoietic stem cell transplantation. Some are already acknowledged as being appropriate treatments for specific indications in the USA.

For example:

1. Chimeric antigen receptor T cell therapy (eg, tisagenlecleucel) is considered an acceptable alternative remission induction therapy to blinatumomab or inotuzumab ozogamicin for patients ≤25 years old with B cell precursor ALL that is refractory or in second or later relapse.

2. Large B cell lymphoma (DLBCL) – for refractory disease or early relapse (<12 months after initial therapy), CD19-directed chimeric antigen receptor (CAR)-T cell therapy using lisocabtagene maraleucel (liso-cel) or axicabtagene ciloleucel (axi-cel), rather than autologous hematopoietic cell transplantation is recommended.

3a. Follicular cell lymphoma in early relapse: for people who are unable to achieve a complete remission (CR), options include several agents
(eg, lenalidomide, tazemetostat, copanlisib) with a plan for autologous hematopietic stem cell transplantation in complete remission or chimeric antigen receptor T cell therapy.

3b. Follicular lymphoma in subsequent relapse: fit patients who attain a CR may proceed with autologous HCT or CAR-T therapy in an attempt to attain long-term remission.

4. Multiple myeloma: for patients with penta-refractory disease, therapies that target BCMA or alkylator-containing regimens rather than other therapies are recommended. BCMA can be targeted using chimeric antigen receptor (CAR)-T cells or the antibody drug conjugate belantamab mafodotin. (Penta-refractory myeloma is defined as myeloma refractory to an anti-CD38 monoclonal antibody (eg, daratumumab, isatuximab), lenalidomide, pomalidomide, bortezomib and arfilzomib).

It is notable that all six FDA-approved CAR T cell therapies target hematologic malignancies. Intense effort is underway to try to mirror their efficacy in solid tumors.

Of note, also, is the frequency and severity of side-effects that they produce, many of which are severe and sometimes fatal. CAR T cell therapies should be administered by hospital physicians experienced in cellular therapy such as allogeneic hematopietic stem cell transplantation.

Allogeneic CAR T cells

The next step for progress is the development of allogeneic universal CAR T cells, which will utilise the T cells of normal volunteer donors and will have additional gene engineering performed on them to minimise the chance of rejection of the CAR T cell and to minimize the risk of GVHD by the CAR T cells before being infused into the recipient. This should markedly reduce the cost of CAR T cell treatment, since one batch of allogeneic CAR T cells will likely serve the needs of a number of recipients.

Finally, the application of CAR T cells for other diseases, particularly solid tumours currently incurable by available treatment such as pancreatic cancer, lung cancer and cancers of the upper alimentary tract, are the subject of much research.

15. ABBREVIATIONS USED

Abbreviations used (other than those explained in Table1, Table 2 and in the FDA label text) are listed below. This list includes abbreviations used in other books in the series Medicine 2020 and the series Modern Medicine 2021.

AC, adriamycin and cyclophosphamide (combination chemotherapy)

ACE, angiotensin-converting-enzyme

ADC, antibody-drug conjugate

ADCC, antibody-dependent cellular cytotoxicity

ADCC, antibody directed enzyme prodrug therapy

AGEP, acute generalized exanthematous pustulosis

AI, aromatase inhibitor

ALK, anaplastic lymphoma kinase

ALL, acute lymphoblastic leukemia

ALT, alanine aminotransferase

AML, acute myeloid leukemia

aPTT, activated partial thromboplastin time

ARR, administration-related reaction

AS, adverse reaction

AS, ankylosing spondylitis

ASCT, autologous stem cell transplant

AST, aspartate aminotransferase

ATA, anti-therapeutic antibody

ATM, ataxia telangiectasia mutated (gene)

AUC, Area Under the Concentration – time curve

AUC (0-inf): AUC curve to infinite time. As we cannot get the assays to go to infinity, we have to extrapolate to infinity. This can be calculated from the AUC(0-t) by the addition of a constant (Clast/λz), where Clast is the last observed quantifiable concentration and λz is the terminal phase rate constant.

BCG, Bacille Calmain-Guerin

BCMA, B cell maturation antigen

BCR-ABL, breakpoint cluster region/Abelson

BCRP, breast cancer resistance protein

b DMARD, biologic disease-modifying anti-rheumatic drug

BRACA1, breast cancer susceptibility gene 1

BTK, Bruton's tyrosine kinase

CAT, cyclophosphamide, adriamycin and taxane (combination chemotherapy)

CDC, complement-dependent cytotoxicity

CDK, cyclin-dependent kinase

C-G, Cockoft-Gault (formula)

cHL, classical Hodgkin Lymphoma

CINV, chemotherapy-induced nausea and vomiting

CIS, carcinoma in situ

CLL, chronic lymphocytic leukemia

Clcr, creatinine clearance rate

CMF, cyclophosphamide, methotrexate, and fluorouracil (combination chemotherapy

CML, chronic myelogenous leukemia (also known as chronic myeloid leukemia)

CPS, combine positive score

CR, complete remission

CRC, colorectal carcinoma

CRISPR, clustered regulatory interspaced short palindromic repeats

CRS, cytokine release syndrome

CS, cytokine storm

csDMARD, synthetic disease-modifying anti-rheumatic drug

CSF1R, colony-stimulating factor receptor 1

CT, computed tomography

CTCAE, Common Terminology Criteria for Adverse Events

CVVHD, continuous veno-venous hemodialysis

DBCL, diffuse B cell lymphoma

DCIS, ductal carcinoma in situ

DFS, disease-free survival

dMMR, deficient mismatch repair

DLBCL, diffuse large B cell lymphoma

DMSO, dimethyl sulfoxide

DPP4, dipeptidyl peptidase-4

DRESS, drug reaction with eosinophilia and systemic symptoms. DRESS syndrome is classified as one form of severe cutaneous adverse reactions (SCARs). In addition to DRESS, SCARs includes four other drug-induced skin reactions, the Stevens–Johnson syndrome (SJS); Toxic epidermal necrolysis (TEN), Stevens–Johnson/toxic epidermal necrolysis overlap syndrome (SJS/TEN)

EBC, early breast cancer

ECG or EKG, electrocardiogram

EFS, event-free durvival

EGF, epidermal growth factor

EGFR, epidermal growth factor receptor

EN, erythema nodosum

ER, estrogen receptor

ET, endocrine therapy

ErbB, derived from erythroblastic leukemia viral oncogene

FBG, fasting blood glucose

FEC, fluorouracil, epirubicin and cyclophosphamide (combination chemotherapy)

FGF, fibroblast growth factor

FGFR, fibroblast growth factor receptor

FISH, fluorescence in situ hybridization

FKBP12/mTOR, FK Binding Protein-12/mammalian target of rapamycin

Flt3, fms like tyrosine kinase 3

FPG, fasting plams glucose

FSH, follicle-stimulating hormone

FU, fluouracil

gBRCAm, BRCA mutated

GBS, Guillain-Barré Syndrome

G-CSF, granulocyte colony-stimulating factor

GD, gestational day

GI, gastro-intestinal

GIST, gastrointestinal stromal tumor

GFR, glomerular filtration rate

GMR, geometric mean ratio

GVHD, graft-versus-host disease

HBV, hepatitis B

HCC, hepatocellular carcinoma

HCV, hepatitis C

HER, human epidermal receptor

HER2, human epidermal growth factor receptor 2

HIV, human immune deficiency virus

HNSCC, head and neck squamous carcinoma

HR, hormone receptor

HRR, homologous recombination repair

HSCT, hematopoietic stem cell transplant

JAK, Janus kinase

KLIFS-3, kinase-ligand interaction fingerprint and structure residue-3

IAP, intra-abdominal pressure

IBC, inflammatory breast cancer

IC, immune cell

ICANS, immune effector cell–associated neurotoxicity syndrome

IFN, interferon

IL, interleukin

ILD, interstitial lung disease

ILN, interstitial lung disease

iNHL, indolent non-Hodgkin lymphoma

IRIS, immune reconstitution inflammatory syndrome

IRR, infusion-related reaction

ITAM, immunoreceptor tyrosine-based activation motif

ITP, idiopathic thrombocytopenic purpura

LBCL, large B cell lymphoma

LCIS, lobular carcinoma in situ

LFT, liver function test

LH, luteinizing hormone

LLN, lower limit of normal

LVEF, left ventricular ejection fraction

Mab, monoclonal antibody

MATE, multi-antimicrobial extrusion protein

MBC, metastatic breast cancer

MCC, Merkel cell carcinoma

mCRPC, metastatic castrate resistant prostate cancer

MEK, mitogen-activated protein kinase

MRI, magnetic resonance imaging

MSI-H, microsatellite instability – high

MUGA, multigated acquisition

NCI-CTC, National Cancer Institute – Clinical Toxicity Criteria

Nib, small i**n**h**ib**itory molecule

NMIBC, non-muscle invasive bladder cancer

NRH, nodular regenerative hyperplasia (of the liver)

NSCLC, non-small cell lung cancer

OHSS, ovarian hyperstimulation syndrome

OS, overall survival

PARP, poly(ADP-ribose) polymerase

PDGF, platelet-derived growth factor

PDGFR, platelet-derived growth factor receptor

PFS, progression-free survival

Ph+, Philadelphia chromosome positive

PI3K, phosphatidylinositol 3-kinase

PI3KA, phosphatidylinositol-4,5-bisphosphate 3-kinase catalytic subunit alpha

PJIA, polyarticular juvenile idiopathic arthritis in patients aged 2 years or older

PJP, *Pneumocystis jiroveci* pneumonia

PK, pharmacokinetic analysis

PKA, protein kinase A

PMBCL, primary mediastinal B cell lymphoma

PML, progressive multifocal leukoencephalopathy

PNET, progressive neuroendocrine tumor (of the pancreas)

PR, progesterone receptor

pRb, retinoblastoma protein

PsA, psoriatic arthritis

PsO, plaque psoriasis

RA, rheumatoid arthritis

RAF, rapidly accelerated fibrosarcoma

RCC, renal cell carcinoma

REMS, Risk Evaluation and Mitigation Strategy

RET, "rearranged during transfection"

ROCK, Rho-associated protein kinase

ROS, 'orphan' receptor tyrosine kinase

rb, retinoblastoma (gene or protein)

r/r, relapsed/refractory

scFv, single-chain Fv fragment

SCARS, severe cutaneous adverse reactions

SCLC, small cell lung cancer

SERD, selective estrogen receptor degrader

SEGA, subependymal giant cell astrocytoma

SIRS, systemic inflammatory response syndrome

SLAM, signalling lymphocytic activation molecule family (CD319)

SJS, Stevens–Johnson syndrome

SLL, small lymphocytic lymphoma

SYK, spleen tyrosine kinase

SWFI, sterile water for injection

TALEN, transcription activator-like effector nuclease

TBC, tuberose sclerosid complex

TCH, docetaxel, carboplatin, and trastuzumab (combination chemotherapy)

TCR, T cell receptor

TEN, toxic epidermal necrolysis

TNBC, triple negative breast cancer

TMB- high, tunor mutational burden - high

TNF, tumor necrosis factor

TRK, tropomyosin receptor kinase

ts DMARD, targeted synthetic disease-modifying anti-rheumatic drug

Tyk, tyrosine-protein kinase

UGT1A1, uridine diphosphate-glucuronosyl transferase 1A1

ULN, upper limit of normal

VEGF, vascular endothelial growth factor

VEGFR, vascular endothelial growth factor receptor

Made in United States
North Haven, CT
04 November 2026

21719221R00146